THE
EVERYTHING®
GUIDE TO A
HEALTHY HOME

Dear Reader,

Ever wonder why so many people seem to be so sick in today's day and age? I do. Especially because I had cancer when I was three years old, and then had fibromyalgia and chronic fatigue syndrome starting in college. These are some pretty major illnesses for anyone, but they all occurred in me before the age of twenty-five. And I am not alone. When modern medicine failed to treat my conditions, I started doing research myself in the quest to be healthy and well again. What I found were shocking and horrifying accounts of what is allowed to be in your home and how these things can affect your health. All of the information is out there in black and white for anyone to find, yet the toxins and health hazards that are now entwined in the average American's life are never reported or talked about. It is possible to protect your health and your family's health without giving up what you love, and I am happy to show you the way. I have done it, and I am here to say that you can, too!

Kimberly Button

Welcome to the EVERYTHING® Series!

These handy, accessible books give you all you need to tackle a difficult project, gain a new hobby, comprehend a fascinating topic, prepare for an exam, or even brush up on something you learned back in school but have since forgotten.

You can choose to read an Everything® book from cover to cover or just pick out the information you want from our four useful boxes: e-questions, e-facts, e-alerts, and e-ssentials.

We give you everything you need to know on the subject, but throw in a lot of fun stuff along the way, too.

We now have more than 400 Everything® books in print, spanning such wide-ranging categories as weddings, pregnancy, cooking, music instruction, foreign language, crafts, pets, New Age, and so much more. When you're done reading them all, you can finally say you know Everything®!

QUESTION

Answers to
common questions

FACT

Important snippets
of information

ALERT

Urgent
warnings

ESSENTIAL

Quick
handy tips

PUBLISHER Karen Cooper

DIRECTOR OF ACQUISITIONS AND INNOVATION Paula Munier

MANAGING EDITOR, EVERYTHING® SERIES Lisa Laing

COPY CHIEF Casey Ebert

ASSISTANT PRODUCTION EDITOR Melanie Cordova

ACQUISITIONS EDITOR Ross Weisman

SENIOR DEVELOPMENT EDITOR Brett Palana-Shanahan

EDITORIAL ASSISTANT Matthew Kane

EVERYTHING® SERIES COVER DESIGNER Erin Alexander

LAYOUT DESIGNERS Erin Dawson, Michelle Roy Kelly, Elisabeth Lariviere, Denise Wallace

Visit the entire Everything® series at *www.everything.com*

THE
EVERYTHING®
GUIDE TO A
HEALTHY HOME

All you need to protect yourself and your family
from hidden household dangers

Kimberly Button

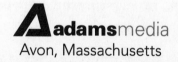

Avon, Massachusetts

To Daniel, for always encouraging me to follow my dreams
and believing that I can achieve them. I love you so much.

To Mom, Dad, and Carrie, for always being proud
of me and for their constant love and support.
Just look at how far I have come!

An Everything® Series Book.
Everything® and everything.com® are registered trademarks of F+W Media, Inc.

Published by Adams Media, a division of F+W Media, Inc.
57 Littlefield Street, Avon, MA 02322 U.S.A.
www.adamsmedia.com

ISBN 10: 1-4405-3057-2
ISBN 13: 978-1-4405-3057-9
eISBN 10: 1-4405-3209-5
eISBN 13: 978-1-4405-3209-2

Printed in the United States of America.

10 9 8 7 6 5 4 3 2 1

Library of Congress Cataloging-in-Publication Data
is available from the publisher.

This publication is designed to provide accurate and authoritative information with regard to the subject matter covered. It is sold with the understanding that the publisher is not engaged in rendering legal, accounting, or other professional advice. If legal advice or other expert assistance is required, the services of a competent professional person should be sought.

—From a *Declaration of Principles* jointly adopted by a Committee of the American Bar Association and a Committee of Publishers and Associations

Many of the designations used by manufacturers and sellers to distinguish their products are claimed as trademarks. Where those designations appear in this book and Adams Media was aware of a trademark claim, the designations have been printed with initial capital letters.

This book is available at quantity discounts for bulk purchases.
For information, please call 1-800-289-0963.

Contents

Acknowledgments

So much of the work that brings to light the shocking hazards that are allowed to be in our homes every day is thanks to the unending efforts of The Environmental Working Group (EWG), a nonprofit organization striving to protect public health. Many thanks to the EWG for supplying easy-to-read research about hard-hitting topics in commonsense terms that we can all understand.

Sincere thanks also goes to the organizations that work relentlessly every day to force policy changes that protect the health and safety of adults and children whom they might never know, but whose well-being they always strive to protect. The resources of Beyond Pesticides, The Campaign for Safe Cosmetics, and Healthy Child Healthy World have provided invaluable research and guidance. Thank you for all that you do.

Top 10 No-Cost Ways to Create a Healthier Home

1. Open your windows and doors. Fresh air from outside will push air polluted with chemicals, allergens, and mold out of your home.

2. Harness the power of the sun. The harsh heat of direct sunlight effectively kills dust mites that live in bedding and upholstery and can cause indoor allergies.

3. Know what is in your water. Each year community water systems must tell you what pollutants, if any, are in your drinking and bath water so you can know what you are exposed to.

4. Reposition your furniture. Move beds and other pieces of furniture on which you spend a lot of time away from electrical power boxes and other places with high EMF fields.

5. Vacuum and sweep regularly. Dust, dirt, allergens, and chemicals settle from the air onto your floor each day, so removing them removes your exposure to the offenders.

6. Kill germs with just soap and water. Viruses, bacteria, and other nasty germs are most effectively killed using simple ingredients instead of hand sanitizers or other harsh chemicals.

7. Clean with ingredients already in your home. Nontoxic food-based ingredients such as vinegar, as well as a common medicine cabinet ingredient such as hydrogen peroxide, can kill germs and remove grime without toxic exposures.

8. Pull weeds and rake leaves. Eliminate the health hazards of yard work by reducing your use of chemical-based lawn products and the toxic fumes of gas-powered lawn equipment.

9. Eliminate and prevent mold. Clean visible mold with detergent and water, and prevent molds from developing by drying spills and leaks as soon as possible.

10. Use a comb and soapy water to kill fleas. Flea-killing products used on your pets and around your home are pesticides that can expose your entire family to unnecessary chemicals.

Introduction

HAVE YOU EVER STOPPED and wondered why everyone seems so sick lately? From soaring obesity, diabetes, and asthma rates to increases in allergies and digestive disturbances, the number of people who have some type of medical complaint certainly feels a lot higher than in previous years. And these are not just minor inconveniences, like the common cold. The health problems facing society today are long-term and life-changing, costing billions of dollars each year and causing emotional harm to countless families.

While there is a great emphasis on eating right and exercising in order to stay healthy and prevent disease, those are not the only answers. Your health is not made up entirely of just what you eat or the amount of activity that you get. The places where you work and live and sleep also comprise a large portion of your health. Your home, workplace, and school can greatly impact your well-being. The quality of air inside these buildings is the very air that you breathe to stay alive each day. The countless surfaces that you touch, from your keyboard to the cutting board, are full of organisms and residues that can end up inside of you. Invisible things like mold and dust mites can be major health offenders. It is time to realize that your home, as well as your homes away from home, are integral pieces of the puzzle of your true health.

People have been living in houses and working in buildings for centuries, though, so what has changed recently that would cause homes to actually be contributing to these major health problems? Along with the modern-day life of the past fifty to a hundred years has come the development of tens of thousands of chemicals that have been created, in theory, for the greater good. These materials are supposed to make your life better, but plenty of studies have shown that they only cause harm. On top of the daily onslaught of chemicals, there's another problem: we just cannot get away from them anymore. Homes are built to prevent less fresh air from coming in, water supplies are tainted with chemical runoffs, and the very items that are applied to your body are often a source of the chemical exposure.

So what's a concerned person to do? Do you have to live a hippie life-style on a commune in order to protect your health? No. Changing your life completely is not the answer. It is not necessary, and, let's face it, it's not practical. But you might want to make some changes. Not big changes, but just some tweaks in the products that you buy and the way that you take care of your home.

Creating a healthier home does not have to be scary, and you do not have to fear the process of cleaning up your exposure to potential toxins. You will not have to give up your lifestyle or even your sense of style to pro-tect your health. Today, there are an astonishing number of nontoxic options that are conveniently available at the places where you shop anyway. You are lucky to be at a pivotal moment in time when it is getting so much easier to choose healthier options for you and your family. It is just a matter of grab-bing for one brand of an item over another.

When trying to create a healthier home, realize that you do not have to do it all. There will be some suggested options that you know just will not work for you. You might try products that are supposed to be healthier for you, but you just don't like how they perform. That's okay. With every posi-tive switch that you do make, you are reducing your exposure to health haz-ards. Even if you do not make the switch now, know that every day there are more and more new products coming available that help you create a nontoxic life, so maybe you will change your thoughts a few months down the road.

You are in control of your health. No one can force you to live an unhealthy life. With every dollar that you spend and with every choice that you make, you make a statement of what is important to you. With this book, you can be empowered to let everyone know that you choose to live healthy and well.

CHAPTER 1

How Healthy Is Your Home?

Your health can be directly related to the health of your home. Sounds crazy? Well, just think about how much time you spend in your home, cooking meals throughout the day, sleeping at night, and relaxing on the weekends. Your home is full of products that you use on a daily basis, from hand soaps to laundry detergent. Your indoor air is full of bits of particles from every material that your home is made of. Your home is not just a structure—it is your very foundation for health.

Redefining the Meaning of Health

Perhaps the health of your home has not exactly been at the top of your concerns. After all, a home is just a building made of wood, bricks, and mortar. If a home is not healthy, does it really matter? You can just buy some new building materials and replace a roof or a floor if there is a problem, right? When it comes to talking about a healthy home, the concern is not for the actual physical structure that you live in; it is for the people who live within the home itself. It turns out that the health of your family is often deeply entwined with the health of your home.

Beyond Eating Right and Exercising

Ask most people what they do to live a healthier life and almost everyone will talk about eating more fruits and vegetables and getting more exercise. Yes, a proper diet and physical activity are essential to a person's health. They should always be part of a healthy lifestyle. But you are much more than just what you eat.

ALERT

People with health problems that are directly related to a product or condition in their home, such as someone who suffers from asthma attacks due to dust mite exposure or eczema due to harsh cleaners, can potentially see a relatively quick and immediate relief from their symptoms with a healthy home change.

There are many more aspects of healthy living other than the food that you put into your body. There is also the air that you breathe, and the products that you apply to be absorbed into your skin, and the water that you ingest. These are all just as important as the food that you choose, yet do not get the same attention or respect. After all, when is the last time that you heard someone boasting about the cleanliness of their water? Have you ever seen a personal trainer who helps you stay on track to improve your indoor air quality?

Short Term versus Long Term

It is easy to focus on health from a nutritional and physical activity standpoint because the results can come so quickly. After eliminating sodas from your diet, you might instantly see a change in your weight on the scale. After walking a mile each day, your waistline can start to become smaller in a matter of weeks. These are all healthy lifestyle changes that can be reinforced because you see results in a relatively short period of time.

Changes to create a healthy home, though, might not exhibit short-term results that you can see. After indulging in too many slices of cake, you will soon see the negative effect on your weight, and you will probably get right back to your healthy eating habits. It is much more difficult to stick with a program of creating a healthier home when you do not see any immediate positive results from making a lifestyle change. Even if you fall off the bandwagon, so to speak, and start bringing products into your once-healthy home that are full of chemicals associated with nasty health risks, you still might not notice a change. That does not mean that damage is not occurring, though, because while food is processed relatively quickly by your body, chemicals are not.

Prevention versus Prescriptions

In today's age of medicine, the focus has been on treating the problem, rather than finding the cause or preventing it from happening in the first place. After all, there seems to be a pill to fix everything, so why worry too much about changing your lifestyle to prevent a problem when you can just medicate later?

FACT

In the United States, 58 percent of nonelderly adults take prescription drugs on a regular basis. For seniors, that number skyrockets to 90 percent. In a ten-year period from 1999 to 2009, the increase in the number of prescriptions that people were purchasing jumped by 39 percent.

Not only do prescription drugs come with a host of side effects that might be worse than the problem that they are designed to treat, but prescriptions can have a serious negative effect on your pocketbook, too. The cost of prescription drugs has increased well above the inflation rate every year over the past decade. With so many people without health insurance, as well as insurance companies that do not adequately cover the cost of prescription drugs, relying on a drug to fix a nongenetic health problem that could have easily been prevented by a lifestyle change is an extremely costly decision.

Causes for Concern

The concept of how your house can affect your health is not an undocumented myth that only a few people believe in anymore. More and more researchers are reporting that often-overlooked and unseen problems, such as mold and dirty indoor air, are causing significant health problems.

Cancer Links

Many of the ingredients and products that are allowed for use in our lives contain known carcinogens, meaning that the ingredients have been scientifically linked to promoting cancer. In May 2010, the President's Cancer Panel stated that "the true burden of environmentally induced cancers has been grossly underestimated" and urged President Barack Obama to "remove carcinogens and other toxins from our food, water, and air that needlessly increase health care costs, cripple our nation's productivity, and devastate American lives."

But it doesn't take a presidential panel to make a vast majority of the country realize that we need to clean up our act in order to live healthier lives. In fact, 83 percent of Americans are worried about the effects of environmental pollution on their family's health, according to the 2006 American Environmental Values Survey by ecoAmerica.

Sick Building Syndrome

There is an actual diagnosis for the health effects that a building can have on a person's health: sick building syndrome. The U.S. Environmental Protection Agency states that sick building syndrome is a term used to "describe situations in which building occupants experience acute health and comfort effects that appear to be linked to time spent in a building, but no specific illness or cause can be identified."

The symptoms of sick building syndrome can be varied, but most often include:

- Dry cough
- Headache
- Eye, nose, and throat irritation
- Skin problems
- Dizziness
- Nausea
- Fatigue
- Problems with concentration
- Odor sensitivity

When an illness can be clinically diagnosed and proven to be contributed directly to a building, it is then called a building-related illness. But asbestos exposure and radon exposure, even though they are a part of the building, are generally not included in the causes of sick building syndrome or building-related illness.

Past Mistakes

In the 1930s and 1940s, lead-based paint was touted as having improved advantages for a child's nursery, hospitals, and schools. Now contractors and educational institutions must use expensive lead-removal techniques to make sure that the neurotoxin cannot accidentally affect a child's health. Asbestos was commonly used because of its wonderful heat-insulating qualities, until it was proven to be linked with cancer. Tobacco was said to help you relax, BPA was added to plastics so that you did not have to be concerned about them breaking, and DDT was sprayed so that humans would not have to deal with pesky insects that could ruin their summertime picnic. Now all of these substances are linked to major health problems.

History has shown that just because a product or ingredient is used does not mean that it is safe. Governments, scientists, and companies all adamantly denied any health harms caused by these products for years and decades, until it was undeniably proven that they do, in fact, cause serious damage. Now millions of families are still dealing with the horrible consequences of exposure to these toxic ingredients.

Celebrities such as Ronald Reagan, Lucille Ball, Babe Ruth, Lou Gehrig, Marlene Dietrich, Joan Crawford, and Jack Webb were all once featured in advertising campaigns in order to help sell cigarettes. Even Santa Claus was once featured in marketing materials for the cigarette brand Pall Mall.

While lead, asbestos, and DDT are just a few examples of substances that had health risks unknown to consumers, these are not the only ones. Not every material ever used has been tested, and many do not stay in commerce long enough to start causing questions about health effects.

Where the Problems Come From

No one purposely goes into a store and buys products that are bad for them. If you knew of the dangers associated with a product, you probably wouldn't buy it. However, because of lax governmental health and safety standards, industry's demand to be unregulated, and marketing practices that are designed to only tell one side of the story, your access to information about the true health and safety of the everyday products in your home is extremely limited.

Misguided Trust

There is an unspoken belief that if a product or service is allowed to be sold to be used on your body or in your home, then it must be safe. Unfortunately, that is often not the case. In the three generations since World War II, more than 80,000 new synthetic, man-made chemicals have been developed for use in products, few of which have been completely tested for safety. Of the nearly 3,000 chemicals that have the highest production volume in the United States, 43 percent have no tests done on basic toxicity and only 7 percent have had complete basic toxicity profiles performed, according to the EPA's Chemical Hazard Availability Study in 1998.

Health and safety testing of ingredients used in household and consumer products is often done by the companies that manufacture the products. The same people who want to sell you something are the same ones who are responsible for saying that it is safe.

Government rules and regulations put the health and safety testing on the shoulders of the businesses, and even after products are put on the market, governmental organizations still do very little health and safety testing on products unless there have been very many complaints.

Misleading Marketing

If a product has the picture of a green leaf on the packaging, is it good for the environment? If your soap states that it is all natural, does that really mean that it is only made from beneficial ingredients created in nature? If nine out of ten dentists recommend a toothpaste, should you just pick up a tube and not even read the label?

ALERT

"Greenwashing" is the term for when companies and advertising agencies mislead the public about the environmentally friendly benefits of a product or service. Greenwashing occurs when you think that a product is healthier on the environment, so you believe that it is healthier for you, too.

Much of the problem with consumers buying products that are not too healthy for them comes from confusing and misleading marketing claims. In today's busy world, not many people have the time to read labels, investigate ingredients, and question a product's safety. Instead, they must rely on what the TV, a billboard, or a flashy magazine or newspaper ad tells them. Unfortunately, the words and images used to promote buying a certain product are almost always unregulated. The terms "hypoallergenic," "natural," and "nontoxic" do not legally mean a thing. Any company can use those words in any way that they see fit without lab tests, health studies, or ingredient reviews being performed.

Have you ever really stood back and watched who is paying for the ads that you are constantly inundated with, from your weather report being sponsored by a local company to the ads that you must look at while sitting on a bus or airplane? You do not find too many ads for fresh fruit or chemical-free cosmetics. Instead, companies with seemingly large purse strings can promote products such as pharmaceuticals, air fresheners, and the latest anti-aging beauty serum. If you really think about the kinds of products and services that are being advertised, so many of them involve chemicals that are cheap to make with synthetic and artificial ingredients that have not been proven to be healthy.

Marketing campaigns also tend to prey on your fears, whether they are warranted or not. For example, some ad campaigns can have you scared silly from possibly being exposed to germs and viruses on every surface of your home. They suggest that unless you buy their disinfectant or cleaning product, you are directly responsible for your family getting sick, so of course you run to the store and buy the product because you want to be a good parent. Unfortunately, there is only an element of truth in those fears. Yes, bacteria and viruses can be bad, but some are actually necessary for good health. There are also chemical-free ways to rid your home from nasty bugs, too, instead of using pricey chemical cleaners. Was the ad campaign wrong? No, but it doesn't tell you the whole truth, either. Marketing agencies know how to push your buttons, so you have to be an educated consumer.

Inexpensive Items

When you are living on a budget, it can be hard to justify sometimes paying a bit more for products made from healthier ingredients. Unfortunately, the simple fact is that ingredients from nature often cost more because they have a limited shelf life and take time and nurturing to grow. Chemicals produced in a lab can be made cheaply, and the low cost of ingredients will result in a lower cost of the final product.

Not all healthy items and ways of living have to be expensive, though. In fact, many healthy lifestyle changes for your home can actually save you money, whether immediately or in the long run. Keep in mind that although many everyday items that you use in your home might be cheap right now, their long-term effects can be quite costly.

FACT

In 2010, organic food sales grew by nearly 8 percent, according to a survey by the Organic Trade Association. Total food sales, which include processed and nonorganic foods, only grew by 0.6 percent in the same year. Organic nonfood items had a nearly 10 percent growth, more than three times the amount of nonorganic items.

New Homes versus Old Homes

Could the type of home that you live in make a big difference in your health? Should you move out of your drafty old home into a brand-new condo to prevent health problems associated with asbestos and mold? Or maybe you are thinking about moving out of a newly built home that you bought a few years ago and into a small farm cottage because of health problems that have start occurring recently. Regardless of where you live, the answers to which kind of home is healthiest are not simple or easy.

New Homes

New homes are constructed of brand-new materials that do not contain known hazards, such as lead and asbestos. Newly installed walls and flooring have a lower risk of containing mold than older homes that have been exposed to much more moisture. With updated health and safety standards, new homes must meet codes that are designed to protect your health.

However, along with the benefits of new homes also come different risks. Starting in the 1970s, new home construction mandated that only five cubic feet per minute of outside air be allowed to enter a home through ventilation. These standards were put into place after an oil shortage in the 1970s to reduce the amount of energy needed to heat and cool a building. Previous standards had called for three times as much outdoor air to be circulated through a building. With less outdoor air circulating through a home, chemicals and pollutants can build up even faster, creating serious indoor air quality problems with new homes.

Building materials themselves can also be a problem. While new building materials do not contain some of the ingredients that have been proven to cause harm, they are still full of new ingredients that have not been tested for long-term health and safety.

FACT

Potential health problems associated with Chinese drywall are just one example of new building materials that might have undocumented health risks. After a building boom between 2004 and 2007 in which Chinese drywall was used extensively, many people started to complain about strong sulfur odors, property damage, and health problems in association with the product.

Whether it is insulation behind the walls or the materials in your flooring and cabinetry, all of the new synthetic products that are used in your home release their fumes into your indoor air. The newer your home is, the more fumes there will likely be, because chemicals used in building materials can off-gas into the air, where small bits of the products will then be breathed in. Off-gassing does not occur indefinitely. Higher concentrations of chemicals are released during the first few months or years that a product has been installed, and then pollutant levels drop over time.

Old Homes

Older homes have probably off-gassed most of their chemical fumes, unless a renovation has recently taken place. Homes built before the mid-1970s also have better air ventilation, which means that you will not breathe in as much nasty stuff. That does not necessarily mean that older homes are healthier, though.

The widespread use of asbestos and lead in older homes means that exposure to these known toxins could be a problem, especially if you have paint that is chipping and peeling or siding that is falling apart. If you want to renovate or start repairing an older home, safety precautions have to be followed in order to prevent toxic exposure.

Older homes can have leaky wood fireplaces that can create carbon monoxide problems. Older plumbing materials used to contain high amounts of lead, which can cause lead exposure through the home's water supply. Extensive years of being subjected to the natural elements and indoor living can cause problems with mold and mildew that might not even be visible. Cracked foundations can further the problem of radon exposure in a home.

Do You Have to Change Your Lifestyle?

Perhaps you agree that there are some questionable things that are allowed to be sold to consumers. You want to create a healthier home, but you are scared that you need to change your life to do it. Don't worry! Creating a healthy home does not mean having to give up the things you love or getting rid of everything you own.

Just Make an Easy Switch

The easiest way to get started on creating a healthy home is just to make some simple switches in items that you might not have that much of an emotional attachment to. For instance, switch out your harmful PVC plastic shower curtain liner for one that looks exactly the same, but is made with a healthier plastic. You can pick up a greener toilet bowl cleaner on your next shopping trip instead of the toxic, chemical-laden kind. Replace or clean an air filter. These are simple things to do that will have a definite impact on the quality of health in your home, yet you probably will not even notice the change.

Shop Where You Want

Choosing healthier products for your home does not mean that you have to change where you shop. Sure, there might be a few things that you need to buy at a specialty store or online, but for the most part, less-toxic versions of everything that you buy can now be found right along with their traditional counterparts. In the grocery store, green cleaners are right beside the conventional cleaners. Mass retailers offer organic bedding options in the same aisle as all of the other bedding. Garden stores usually have a section with organic fertilizers. Pet stores sell natural treats and chemical-free shampoos. Whatever aspect of your life that you want to buy a healthier product for, you can usually easily find it in major stores.

Shopping online is also a great way to stock up on nontoxic options without having to drive to stores on the other side of town or change your routine. At any time of the day, you can hop online and either have healthier options added to stores that you buy products from anyway, such as Amazon.com, or purchase from small specialty retailers that might not have the money to start a brick-and-mortar store with fancy advertising but who sell quality products nonetheless.

Inspiring Future Changes

With every small step that you take to choose a nontoxic product over another, you will come to see that it is not hard or complicated to create a healthy home for you and your family. Small steps can lead to larger ones when you see the results of a positive change. After successfully switching hand soaps, you might be inspired to switch your shampoo, too. When you see how much healthier your hair and skin look with a shower filter, you might be encouraged to install a kitchen sink water filter, as well.

You Don't Have to Do It All

Keep in mind that you do not have to make every healthy change possible. Some of the changes you might just not be able to do, such as removing carpet or buying only solid wood furniture. Other changes you might try hard to do, but you just don't seem to have much success. It is okay to not change your life completely. After all, everyone has special circumstances in their own lives. With every change that you make, though, the amount of chemicals and toxins that your body has to process will diminish, resulting in a healthier lifestyle for you and your family.

CHAPTER 2

Common Household Dangers

There are a few serious health hazards that can affect everyone in their home, regardless of where you live or how clean your house is. The scary thing is that these common problems are usually undetectable by taste, smell, or sight. You have got to know about the hazard first in order to protect yourself from it. With some easy-to-follow guidelines, though, you can protect your family from major health offenders and rest a little easier in your home.

Mold

Mold is not just a cosmetic problem in your shower. Mold can be very damaging to your health and can lurk in places that you can't see and do not think about. This naturally occurring substance can start to grow on carpet, drywall, insulation, and wood behind the walls. Even if you do not see telltale black spots of mold that you might be familiar with in your shower, mold can be lurking throughout your house.

Controlling Mold

Mold is a fungus whose spores exist in everyone's home, floating through the air. But mold, also known as mildew, does not start to grow and thrive unless it has moisture. That is where the problem lies, but that is also the opportunity to control it. You can take proper precautions to halt mold growth before it has a chance to become a problem.

The simple solution is to reduce the dampness and moisture problems that you might have in your home, ranging from piles of wet towels on the bathroom floor to plumbing leaks in the kitchen and around your home. Clean up and dry out leaks, spills, and other moisture problems as soon as possible, ideally within two days. Fix leaks in your plumbing system and toilet. Remove standing sources of water, like drip trays under the refrigerator or air conditioner, to reduce the amount of humidity and potential sources for mold growth. Wipe off condensation that might be developing on the inside of your windows, on the walls, and on pipes.

ESSENTIAL

If you need to control the moisture problems inside your home, buy a dehumidifier. The appliance will automatically regulate the moisture levels and pull moisture out of your indoor air when necessary. You will want to keep your indoor air humidity low, around a 30–50 percent relative humidity and not above 60 percent, in order to control mold growth.

Proper air flow can also prevent mold growth, by allowing any spots with moisture to naturally dry out. Allow ventilation to occur between furniture and the walls to avoid moisture collecting in drywall materials. Ceiling fans will increase air circulation and ventilation, while also helping to dry out moisture. Have a musty closet? Open closet doors to allow for air circulation. Always use your ventilation fan when taking a shower and cooking in the kitchen, but make sure that the fan vents to outside of your home, and not somewhere else inside. If you do not have a ventilation fan, open the windows when possible to let the heat and humidity escape. Depending on the time of year, open your windows, run the air conditioner or heat, or turn on the dehumidifier if you have one, to reduce your home's humidity levels.

Mold growth does not just start inside the home, it can also be caused by outside problems, too. Make sure that your lawn sprinklers do not spray directly onto your house, which just increases the amount of water that can seep inside. If your gutters are clogged with leaves and debris, clean them out and repair them to prevent water from pooling on the roof and near your foundation. Grade the ground so that water flows away from your house to prevent water seeping in through the foundation.

Mold and Your Health

Mold can really wreak havoc on some people's health. Molds actually produce allergens, so mold can cause allergic reactions, such as hay fever–type symptoms such as sneezing, runny nose, red eyes, and a skin rash. Mold can act as an irritant to your eyes, skin, nose, throat, and lungs. It can be a contributing factor in chronic upper respiratory problems, and mold can cause asthma attacks in people with asthma who are allergic to mold. In some cases, mold can produce substances called mycotoxins that can have toxic health effects.

How to Get Rid of Mold

Can you spot mold on a surface in your house? To kill mold, clean non-porous surfaces with detergent and water, not bleach. Bleach is not as effective at killing mold as many believe. You can also add a few drops of tea tree oil into a spray bottle of water and spray on the surface to effectively clean the surface and kill the mold.

For mold growing on fabrics, wash the item in hot water with detergent. For even more mold-killing power, allow it to dry in the hot sun. Mold growing in porous materials, such as drywall or other building materials, might need to be replaced instead of cleaned. If mold reappears after you have thoroughly cleaned the surface with detergents and you are controlling moisture levels, you need to look into options for removal. For large patches of mold, greater than ten square feet, it is best to consult a professional.

When cleaning or removing mold, it is essential to protect yourself from inhaling the spores. Wear a mask that is designed to prevent mold inhalation. A cheap and flimsy face mask will not protect you from inhaling mold spores that are disrupted in the cleaning process. Goggles can prevent mold spores from getting into your eyes, too, but be sure there are no ventilation holes in the goggles, or else mold can still enter.

Lead

The danger of lead in children's toys is often talked about when there is a toy recall, but did you know that the most significant source of lead poisoning for people of all ages is in materials that might already be in your home? While lead exposure is especially problematic for children, lead is not something that you want to expose yourself to, no matter your age.

FACT

A great resource for information on lead is the National Lead Information Center (*www.epa.gov/lead/nlic.htm*). You can order up to fifteen documents free of charge from their vast library on lead-related topics (*www.epa.gov/opptintr/lead/pubs/nlic.htm*). Lead information specialists are also available to talk by phone at (800) 424-LEAD or communicate through e-mail.

Lead is all natural. It is a metal found in the earth's crust. But just because something exists in nature doesn't necessarily make it safe for you to be exposed to. Lead is a highly toxic metal, but because it is cheap and readily available, it is unfortunately used in many household products.

Many Health Dangers of Lead

Lead exposure is a serious problem with serious health consequences, yet the dangers are not widely known. To make matters worse, lead is not something that you can smell or see or taste. Lead is most often associated with problems of the central nervous system, including:

- Hyperactivity
- Inattentiveness
- Lower IQ levels
- Irritability
- Difficulties with learning and reading
- Shortened attention spans
- Delays in physical and mental development

Lead does not just affect the brain, though. While the health effects of lead on a child's developing nervous system are most often talked about, lead can have other health effects in both children and adults, including:

- Muscle and joint pain
- Kidney problems
- Fatigue and irritability
- Hearing loss
- Seizures
- Nausea
- Constipation
- Abnormal and reduced sperm
- Miscarriages
- Anemia
- Hypertension

More than one million children in the United States have lead paint poisoning, according to the EPA. Lead levels can be measured in your blood, so a simple blood test can tell you whether or not you or your children have already been exposed to high amounts of lead. Young children up to two years old should be tested for lead, as well as anyone who has been exposed to lead hazards.

Lead-Based Paints

If you live in a home built before 1978, then you could be at risk for lead exposure. Lead was often used in paint until 1978, when it was finally banned after determining the harmful health effects. Lead doesn't just disappear, though. It does not escape into the atmosphere over time. No, lead stays put where it is. So if any portion of your home still has remnants of old lead-based paint, you could be at risk, especially if you are planning a renovation.

But don't worry too much yet. Lead-based paint is considered relatively safe unless it starts peeling or chipping. When that starts to happen, the paint can become lead-based dust and enters your indoor air, where you inhale it. To take proper precautions, take a look throughout your home if it was built before 1978—both inside and out—to spot any peeling or chipping paint. This includes the inside of door jambs and windows, where constant opening and scraping can start to chip off paint. If you have no wear and tear, that is great! If you do have some problem areas, you will want to take proper precautions. You can carefully wipe up areas of chipping and peeling paint with a damp cloth for removal. Never sand or scrape lead-based paint, as the dust generated will be inhaled and will contain lead. Wear a ventilation mask while cleaning the area.

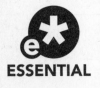
ESSENTIAL

To properly clean lead-containing dust, use a mixture of warm water and powdered automatic dishwasher detergent containing phosphates, since most cleaners will not remove lead. (Note: Most green cleaners do not contain phosphates, so you might need to borrow some from a neighbor who hasn't quite made the green switch yet.)

If you think that you might have lead-based paint still in your home, and you want to remove it or undergo a renovation, it is important to hire a professional with experience and certifications in removing lead-based paint and in testing for lead. Contractors are now required by the EPA to be Lead-Safe Certified if working with lead-based paint in homes, schools, and child care facilities built before 1978, so check your contractor's certifications. The EPA has a search engine (*http://cfpub.epa.gov/flpp/searchrrp_firm.htm*) where you can find EPA-certified renovation firms.

During a renovation of an older home that could contain lead, it is vitally important to take the proper precautions and to relocate to another area where lead-based dust cannot enter. Be sure that the entire area is properly cleaned before you are allowed access back into the site. If you live in an older home that recently underwent a renovation and proper precautions were not taken regarding lead-based paint, consider having a blood test for lead poisoning, especially in young children.

ALERT

Old painted furniture might contain lead-based paint, too. Keep an eye on furniture painted before 1978 for any chipping and peeling. You will want to pay special attention to family heirloom furniture pieces, such as cribs and rocking chairs that might still contain lead-based paint and are used in children's rooms.

Other Places Where Lead Lurks

Lead can also find its way into your home through your water (see Chapter 4 for more discussion on the topic). Public water systems test for lead, so there is not as big of a risk from that source of water. The problem, however, could lie with your home's individual plumbing if it includes materials made with lead. The only way to know for sure is to have your home water quality tested for lead.

The dirt on the bottom of your shoes can also unknowingly bring lead into your home. Soil outside of buildings that have been painted with a lead-based paint can contain residues of lead, as does soil from roadsides that have accumulated years of exhaust from cars using leaded gas. To prevent lead from being tracked inside your home, purchase doormats for every entrance into your house, and make sure that every family member wipes their feet on the mat when entering. Even better, remove your shoes before entering the house. Do not let children or pets play in soil that could contain lead, either.

Lead can also be found in leaded crystal and lead-glazed pottery. Keep this in mind when choosing new pieces and avoid storing food or drink in any product that might contain lead.

Radon

Radon is the second leading cause of lung cancer in the United States, just behind cigarette smoking. Each year, radon is thought to kill more people through lung cancer than the amount of traffic fatalities caused by drunk driving. Lung cancer is the only known human health effect from air-based radon exposure. Radon is a serious health risk, yet one that can easily be prevented.

ESSENTIAL

You can download many publications regarding radon, including testing for radon before buying or selling a home, on the EPA's website (*www.epa.gov/radon/pubs/index.html*). Some of the publications are available in print form and can be ordered for free through the EPA's National Service Center for Environmental Publications (*www.epa.gov/nscep/*). The National Radon Hotline, (800) SOS-RADON, has a staff that answers consumer questions.

What Is Radon?

Radon occurs naturally in the earth. It is a radioactive gas that is created when uranium breaks down. It is most often found in igneous rock and soil. As a radioactive gas, radon is a known carcinogen, which means it causes cancer. Because radon cannot be seen, smelled, or tasted, it is difficult to know where radon is unless you test for it.

In the United States, radon can be found in all fifty states. Some areas of the country have higher radon levels than others. The EPA has a map of radon zones (*www.epa.gov/radon/zonemap.html*) for the entire nation based on predicted average indoor radon screening levels. The same information can also be found for individual states (*www.epa.gov/radon/where youlive.html*) with estimated radon levels broken down by county.

Radon Exposure at Home

Radon can be found naturally occurring in soil, rock, or water. A home built on top of soil that contains radon will have a lower air pressure inside the home than the air pressure that is found within the soil. This difference in pressure creates a vacuum-like effect, with air being drawn inside the home from outside. Along with the air being drawn into the home through cracks and openings in the foundation, radon can also enter, as well. Radon levels tend to be highest in basements and other areas of the home that are below grade or in direct contact with the soil.

Radon can also enter your home through water. The gas can be released through the water when you shower and radon escapes through the steam. Some materials used in the home, such as granite countertops, can also have small amounts of radon. In the grand scheme of things, though, your radon exposure from water and building materials is minimal compare to radon exposure through the air.

According to the EPA, the average amount of radon found in American homes is 1.3 picocuries per liter (pCi/L). Outdoor concentrations typically average 0.4 pCi/L. At 4 pCi/L or higher within a home, the EPA recommends that the home be modified to reduce radon levels. While the EPA has safety limits of radon level exposure, it is important to realize that the EPA has stated "there is no known safe level of exposure to radon," and suggests reducing radon levels in your home even if they are below 4pCi/L.

Testing for Radon

The only way to know for sure if your home has radon is to test for it. The EPA, the Surgeon General, the American Lung Association, the American Medical Association, and the National Safety Council, among others, have all stressed that testing for radon is important to create a healthy home.

Testing for radon is relatively simple and quite affordable, and test kits are readily available. There are two different types of radon tests, both short-term and long-term. Short-term test kits, which test the air inside your home from a few days to three months, tell you quickly whether you might have a radon problem that needs to be fixed. The kits can alert you to whether there might be a problem that you need to investigate further by testing again or contacting a radon professional. Long-term tests, which are designed to track the radon levels in your home for more than three months, will give you a better idea of what your home's radon levels actually are over the course of a year. Radon test kits can be purchased online, at home improvement stores, or at mass retailers. Kansas State University's National Radon Program Services (*http://sosradon.org/test-kits*), which is funded by the EPA, sells affordable short-term test kits for $15 and long-term test kits for $25. Some state health departments might offer low-cost or free radon test kits, as well. The EPA has a listing of state radon offices (*www.epa.gov/radon/whereyoulive.html*) to help you find whom to contact.

If you would rather hire a professional to test your home for radon, or you need to find a professional to mitigate a known radon problem, the National Radon Safety Board (*www.nrsb.org*) and the National Environmental Health Association's National Radon Proficiency Program (*www.neha-nrpp.org*) both have search engines to find a certified radon professional where you live. You can also contact your state's radon office (*www.epa.gov/radon/whereyoulive.html*) for a list of professionals in your state.

What to Do If You Have Radon

If you do find elevated levels of radon in your home, rest assured that there is a way to fix the problem. You do not have to move out of your home. Many radon remediation techniques can reduce the levels of radon up to 99 percent and might not be as expensive as you would think.

ESSENTIAL

Opening the windows of your home to increase ventilation can decrease the radon levels inside your home. However, once the home is closed up again, with the windows and doors closed, the radon levels will return to their previous levels in twelve hours or less.

There are many different ways to prevent radon from accumulating to high levels in your home. The technique that is used depends on the type of foundation that your home has, such as a basement, slab-on-grade, or crawl space, as well as other concerns regarding your specific home and where you live. All the techniques follow one of two methods to reduce radon levels—either prevent radon from entering in the first place, or reduce the levels that are already in the house.

If you have a private well and radon is found in your water, you can purchase devices to remove the radon from your water. Radon can be found in public water systems, too, in which case you would need to contact your water supplier for more information or invest in a filter to remove radon from your home's water.

Carbon Monoxide

You can't see it. You can't smell it. You can't taste it. If you are exposed to it, though, carbon monoxide can immediately make you feel very ill or even kill you. It is a dangerous gas that can accumulate in homes, which is why it is essential to know where it can come from and how to detect it.

Carbon monoxide is produced from the incomplete burning of fuel. Anything that runs off of coal, wood, oil, kerosene, charcoal, natural gas, or propane can potentially create carbon monoxide. Portable generators and cars can create carbon monoxide, too, because of their internal combustion engines.

Automobile Exhaust

Maybe you are familiar with the toxic effects of carbon monoxide poisoning due to mystery movies in which someone dies in a closed garage after inhaling too much carbon monoxide from a running car. Yes, carbon monoxide from automobile exhaust is one of the main sources of the harmful gas, and it can be a very real concern at your home.

If you have an attached garage, one that shares a wall with another room in your house, never let a car idle inside. Even if the garage doors are open, dangerous amounts of carbon monoxide can still build up inside and migrate indoors into other rooms of your house.

Heating and Cooking

Certain heating systems can cause carbon monoxide poisoning inside your home. Unvented gas and kerosene space heaters can allow carbon monoxide poisoning to build up in the rooms in which they are used. Furnaces, chimneys, and wood stoves can all cause carbon monoxide exposure, too, if there is any buildup preventing the gas from escaping or a back draft in the system. Gas ovens that you cook with can also be a source of carbon monoxide exposure, as well as gas water heaters and gas dryers.

Whether a heating or cooking appliance, it is always necessary to have proper ventilation when using the product. For gas stoves, use an exhaust fan when cooking to capture carbon monoxide and other gases. It is important, however, that the fan vents to the outdoors and not to another area in your home. For heating systems, make sure that you have adequate ventilation in association with the appliance and open the flues when using a fireplace. For unvented gas and kerosene space heaters, always open the door to the room where they are being used and have a window open a couple of inches somewhere in the house. Never sleep in a room with an unvented gas or kerosene heater.

Professional installation, proper maintenance, and regular inspections are also key to making sure that your system is not damaged in any way and will not produce high amounts of carbon monoxide. If you see damage, or suspect that there might be a problem, always play it safe and consult a professional.

Portable Generators

A major reason for many lethal carbon monoxide poisonings is operating a portable generator indoors. Portable generators are great during times of a power outage, but these devices can create high amounts of carbon monoxide that can quickly escalate to fatal levels. Amidst the severe weather of the busy 2005 hurricane season, which included Hurricane Katrina, at least ninety-four people died because of generator-related carbon monoxide poisonings, according to the U.S. Consumer Product Safety Commission (CPSC).

Even with the windows open or the garage or basement door open wide, generators should never, ever be used indoors because of the dangerous gases that can accumulate. Even outdoors, you must be careful about how close a generator is operated near your house. Always use a generator far enough away from your home, garage, or other structure that gases cannot enter the building.

ALERT

Charcoal is often used in times of power outages for heating and cooking, too. Charcoal can emit high levels of carbon monoxide in enclosed spaces. Never use charcoal to cook on a grill in your home, garage, or basement. Charcoal should never be used in a fireplace or wood stove, either.

Know the Warning Signs

Because carbon monoxide is so hard to detect, it is imperative to know the warning signs of carbon monoxide poisoning so that you know when to get help. Recognizing the symptoms might be your only indication that you have a carbon monoxide problem. Low levels of carbon monoxide can cause fatigue, headaches, shortness of breath, and chest pain. More moderate levels of carbon monoxide can cause symptoms such as:

- Severe headaches
- Dizziness
- Nausea
- Fainting
- Vision problems
- Mental confusion and disorientation
- Flu-like symptoms

Carbon monoxide detectors are a good way to alert you to dangerous levels of carbon monoxide in your home, but they are not foolproof. It is always advisable to have several carbon monoxide detectors throughout your home, especially near bedrooms. But carbon monoxide detectors do not work nearly as well as smoke detectors. Laboratory testing has shown varying degrees of protection, but technology is still improving to make the detectors more reliable. When purchasing a carbon monoxide detector, look for a brand that has been certified by Underwriters Laboratories.

If a carbon monoxide detector goes off, or if you notice symptoms of carbon monoxide poisoning, immediately get out of your house and get access to fresh air. Do not try to go through your home and figure out where the carbon monoxide might be coming from, because the gases could become even more dangerous the longer that you stay in the building. If you suspect that your carbon monoxide detector set off an alarm unnecessarily, first make sure that no one is exhibiting any signs of carbon monoxide exposure. If no one feels any health effects, open your windows to ventilate the house and then turn off combustion appliances while determining whether the alarm was warranted or not.

CHECKLIST TO CONTROL COMMON HOUSEHOLD DANGERS

❑ Look through your house to find and remove sources of moisture. This is one of the most important ways to prevent mold growth before it compromises your indoor air.

❑ Take proper precautions to clean up and remove lead-based paint from before 1978. Lead in paint is the most common source of lead exposure for children and adults. Removing the paint before it can become dust reduces your risk of inhaling lead.

❑ Use a home test kit to find out if your home has radon. A simple kit can give you accurate readings about this potentially harmful gas in your home.

❑ Purchase a carbon monoxide detector for use in your home. An indoor detector is often the only way to know if this colorless, odorless gas is present at dangerous levels.

❑ Get a blood test to check for lead levels if you might have had high exposure to lead. Especially important for children, a blood test can let you quickly know if there is too much lead in your system.

❑ Do not let a car idle in the garage, even if the doors are open. Carbon monoxide can rapidly build up in a garage, even with ventilation.

❑ Clean and remove mold with detergent and water, not bleach. Bleach will not effectively kill all mold, but detergent is highly effective at killing the indoor air polluter.

❑ Never use a portable generator or portable cooking device inside your garage or in your home. Carbon monoxide levels are especially high around portable cooking devices and should never be used in enclosed spaces.

CHAPTER 3

Indoor Air Quality

You spend a lot more time indoors nowadays than your grandparents did two generations ago. That's not good for many reasons, but most importantly, too much time indoors can be really bad for your health. Indoor air is surprisingly more polluted than outdoor air. Not just a little more polluted, but a lot! With every breath you take, your body has to filter out the stuff that accumulates in your indoor air. One of the first steps to take in creating a healthy home is to clean up your air.

The Problem with Indoor Air

Indoor air pollution levels can be up to five times higher than pollution levels outside. Even worse, the average American spends 90 percent of their time indoors. That means that nine out of every ten breaths that you take each and every day, you are inhaling heavily polluted indoor air that might be full of not-so-healthy particles.

Your Air and Your Health

Think that indoor air quality is not a big problem? It is. Poor indoor air is increasingly being tied to allergy problems and asthma, either as the cause or as a source of flareups. The American Lung Association and the EPA, among others, have voiced great concern about the effect of poor indoor air on the quality of the nation's health. Since one in fifteen Americans have asthma, and many, many more have allergies, that is a big deal.

But there are even more health risks, too. Among the short-term health effects from poor indoor air are:

- Headaches
- Fatigue
- Dizziness
- Nausea
- Eye, nose, and throat irritation
- Memory impairment
- Visual disorders

There are long-term health risks from exposure to polluted air, too, though they are not as well researched. Respiratory problems, cancer, heart disease, and damage to the liver, kidney, and central nervous system can be caused by exposure to chemicals that can accumulate in the air.

Perhaps you have unknowingly experienced the health effects of poor indoor air quality. Do you feel worse at work than you do at home? Do you feel better at work than you do at home? Have you ever entered a store or someone else's house and noticed a weird smell that gave you a headache or just made you feel not quite right? These symptoms are not just all in your head. They are real, and they can be attributed to indoor air quality.

FACT

You can speak with someone directly at the American Lung Association about lung health and air quality topics, including allergies, asthma, smoking, lung cancer, and environmental health. Call (800) 548-8252 to speak to a registered nurse or registered respiratory therapist, or use the online features (*www.lungusa.org/about-us/lung-helpline.html*) to chat or e-mail a question.

Volatile Organic Compounds

So, why can indoor air be so nasty? Some of the main culprits are volatile organic compounds (VOCs). Do not let the word "organic" fool you into thinking these substances are healthy. VOCs are really tiny particles of chemicals that come unattached from a product over time and are emitted as gases. It is also known as off-gassing. Off-gassing occurs from both solid and liquid items. Among the top VOC offenders, depending on what materials the product is made from, are:

- Carpeting
- Paints and painting supplies
- Cleaning supplies
- Aerosol sprays
- Furniture
- Building supplies
- Fuels
- Pesticides
- Hobby materials, such as glues and adhesives
- Copiers and printers

ALERT

Some things that you do at home that involve products with high VOC levels can dramatically and quickly decrease the quality of your home's indoor air. The EPA has found that certain activities, such as paint stripping, can spike the levels of some VOCs up to 1,000 times normal outdoor levels and remain that way for several hours.

The more synthetic and chemical-based products used in the building of your house, your décor, and everyday use, the greater the concentration of VOCs that will likely start building up in your indoor air.

Other Indoor Air Contaminants

VOCs are not the only culprit for poor indoor air quality, though. Everyday life can contribute to the pollution problem inside your own four walls. Particulates from cleaning products, burning candles, and tiny remnants from perfumes and hair sprays also build up over time, regardless of how synthetic or natural the ingredients might be. Little bits of grease from sautéing vegetables for dinner and smoke from that last cooking accident circulate through your entire home. Even naturally occurring problems such as animal dander, pollen, mold, and mildew can further the problem of polluted indoor air.

Lack of Ventilation

The desire to have more energy-efficient houses is ironically a contributing factor behind poor indoor air quality. Because most homes made after the 1970s, and especially newer homes, are more air-tight and well-sealed to prevent heating and cooling loss, there is less of an exchange of fresh air from outside to replace the stagnant air inside. Unless you install a proper air filtration system in your home, or frequently open the windows and doors, you might not be getting much fresh air into your home to replace the bad air.

Dust and Dust Mites

Perhaps you have heard of dust mites before, perhaps not. They are not really something that people like to talk about. But here is the thing—nearly every single home has dust mites, no matter how clean or how dirty your house is. Dust mites live in dust, which constantly circulates through your home's indoor air. These creatures, which can't be seen by the naked eye, can cause some major health problems that might otherwise be blamed on other health conditions.

What Are Dust Mites?

Dust mites are microscopic creatures—smaller than $\frac{1}{70}$ of an inch—that thrive on sloughed-off human and animal skin. They do not bite or get under your skin, but they are still there on surfaces where you sit and sleep. These small creatures feed on the nearly $\frac{1}{5}$ of an ounce of dead skin that you naturally slough off each week. If you have furry pets, then dust mites are definitely feeding off of the pet dander and skin that your pet sheds.

Where Do They Live?

Since dust mites live on shed human skin and animal dander, they will be found in places where there is an accumulation of that type of debris, such as in bedding and on upholstered furniture. Dust can contain the debris of animal dander and skin, too, so any place that accumulates dust will harbor dust mites, hence the name.

FACT

It has been estimated that a typical used mattress can contain between 100,000 to 10 million dust mites, both dead and alive, inside. A two-year-old pillow can attribute approximately 10 percent of its weight to dead dust mites and their droppings that accumulate in the materials.

Dust mites thrive in warm weather, typically around 75 to 80 degrees, which is roughly where your home's thermostat is probably set to in both summer and winter. Dust mites especially enjoy high humidity, such as 70–80 percent relative humidity. Fabrics and upholstery can retain moisture, whether from the ambient air or perspiration from you, on which dust mites thrive, so you will likely find dust mites in curtains, bedspreads, pillows, and other upholstered items that you might not think about.

Allergic Reactions

These little creatures can pack a big punch when it comes to affecting your health. Dust mites can cause allergy problems, many of which are attributed to vague "indoor allergies" when they could really just be "dust mite allergies." Surprisingly, dust mite allergies are not allergies to the actual pest, but its feces. Disgusting, for sure. Exposure to dust mites and their droppings creates a significant risk factor for health problems such as:

- Sneezing
- Itchy, watery eyes
- Runny nose
- Nasal stuffiness
- Stuffy ears
- Respiratory problems
- Eczema
- Asthma

Killing Dust Mites

Dust mites are nasty and their health effects aren't nice, so how do you get rid of them? It is quite simple, really. Lower humidity levels and proper cleaning are just about all you need to rein these suckers in and create a healthier house. Before you start controlling the future growth of dust mites in your home, though, you have to kill the existing ones first. Start by washing your bedding—all of your bedding. This includes your sheets, the blankets, the comforter, the pillowcases, the sham covers, the dust ruffle, and anything else fluffy and upholstered that you keep on your bed. Hot water (at least 140 degrees Fahrenheit) will kill dust mites. While you are at it, you might want to throw in any cloth curtains throughout your home, too, if they can be washed. Blankets and pillows stored in the closets or located in the family room also need a thorough cleaning.

Dust mites can take harbor in items that you cannot put in the washing machine, such as mattresses, rugs, pillows, decorative bedding, upholstered furniture, and even your floor's carpeting. For these items, place them in direct sunlight outside for a few hours if possible. The heat of the sun's rays will kill dust mites. Freezing temperatures work, too, in the middle of winter. If you cannot place them outside, vacuum or beat the dust out of the items as much as possible. You can also use a steam cleaner to kill dust mites with the high heat of the water vapor. Just be sure that you are able to thoroughly dry the item or else you might have a mold problem.

To get rid of dust mites, you also have to get rid of dust. Go through your entire home and dust with a wet cloth, instead of dry dusting, to capture as much dust as possible. Wipe off blinds and other window coverings. Clear the clutter throughout your home, as it is hard to dust around lots of objects, and piles of stuff are great at accumulating dust.

FACT

Stuffed toys, whether they are a pet's or a child's, can harbor dust mites. Wash the toys in hot water and leave lying in the sun for a few hours, or put in a plastic zip-top bag and place inside the freezer for a few hours. Be sure to shake out the toys afterward.

Once you have gone through and cleaned everything, now is the time to limit the amount of dust mites that can exist in your home. When you reduce the humidity in your home, dust mites are killed off. Use a gadget called a hygrometer, which is often found on many indoor weather stations, to monitor the humidity levels inside your home and take appropriate action when needed. Run your air-conditioning during warm weather to keep humidity at bay or use a dehumidifier. Dust and vacuum frequently. Wash your bedding in hot water at least once a week. Items such as comforters and bed ruffles can be washed less frequently if you are now controlling dust mite growth.

Heating Systems

There are many ways to keep your home comfortably warm in the winter, but a lot of the methods can create poor indoor air quality. Many heaters are combustion sources that are known to cause indoor air pollution. Combustion sources are products that burn fuels, which can either be a gas, a liquid, or a solid. Furnaces, space heaters, fireplaces, wood stoves, and gas stoves that burn fuels such as oil, gas, kerosene, coal, and wood are considered combustion sources.

Dangerous Gases

Among the most dangerous gases that can build up in your home from using combustion source heaters are carbon monoxide and nitrogen dioxide. As discussed in earlier in this book, carbon monoxide is a colorless, odorless gas that can cause flu-like symptoms, as well as headaches, dizziness, confusion, disorientation, and fatigue. Unlike carbon dioxide, nitrogen dioxide can be smelled and might be seen as a reddish-brown gas. Linked with respiratory illnesses and especially problematic to asthmatics, nitrogen dioxide can affect the mucous membranes of your eyes, nose, and throat.

Safety Precautions

If you have a furnace, chimney, or flue, make sure that you have an annual inspection to check that everything is in proper working order and vented appropriately. You should regularly look for cracks, built-up debris, and other damage to the area that could cause a problem. Follow the maintenance instructions that came with your system. Be sure to change the filters regularly, either according to your manufacturer's directions, or at least every couple of months.

If you use an unvented space heater that runs off of gas or kerosene, you must pay special attention to the fumes that can build up indoors. The EPA suggests keeping a door open to the room where the heater is operating so that fumes do not build up in the room. It is also advised to open a window slightly to allow fresh air in and gases to escape.

ESSENTIAL

A yellow-tipped flame in a gas space heater or stove is often a sign that many pollutants are being emitted. If the yellow-tipped flame occurs for a length of time, you may need to adjust the settings on the heater or stove until you have a flame with a blue tip.

Fireplaces and wood stoves can cause dangerous gases to accumulate in your home, too, but there is another health hazard associated with these heating systems. Small particles, such as ash, can be released into the air when burning wood and other solid fuels. The particles can then be inhaled and carried into your lungs, where they can damage the lung tissue. Never burn pressure-treated wood because it is made with chemicals that should not be released into your indoor air and inhaled.

Air Fresheners

If you believe the commercials that frequently populate the airwaves, air fresheners can make your whole home smell like a bed of roses. They will make your family happy and your dog smell good, and you can leave rotten fish and meat in your trash for days on end. Your need to do any and all housework suddenly vanishes when you own an air freshener, and your house will be the social hub of the neighborhood. Think again.

Take Care of the Actual Problem First

Air fresheners have been designed to cover up the odor of chores that need to be done. Rotten meat will smell when it decomposes. Moldy smells indicate a mold problem. Stinky gym shoes need to be washed. No amount of air freshening products will change these simple facts.

If you find yourself always buying an air freshener or if you have one always plugged in several rooms of the house, consider why you are using them. Do you simply like the smell of fragrance throughout the home? Or are you trying to cover the odor of a problem? If you are trying to cover up a foul odor, you would probably be better off taking care of the problem for many health and safety reasons. Dogs need to be bathed, not only for odor control, but also for basic health and hygiene issues. Diapers need to be thrown out regularly, considering the waste that is in them! A funky smell coming from the vents in a certain room of your house needs to be investigated to make sure it is not a serious health hazard.

What Makes the Smell

A majority of air fresheners on the market today use artificial or synthetic fragrances in the product to give off a certain smell. After all, it is hard to actually capture the natural essence of a "summer rain" or "sunny day" smell, isn't it? The term "artificial fragrance" is not just one chemical used to scent a product. Fragrance is a generic term that is used to identify the presence of up to 3,194 ingredients that have been blended together to make one scent. Under consumer pressure, the International Fragrance Association has finally released their "Ingredients" list (*www.ifraorg.org/en-us/Ingredients_2*), and it contains a mind-boggling amount of materials that can be used to create a fragrance. You have no idea what chemicals have been used to create an "artificial fragrance," and by law, the manufacturers do not have to tell you. Yet consumers willingly pollute their indoor air with these unknown offenders on a daily basis.

FACT

More than eighty-nine contaminants were found in a popular air freshener brand in a study by the Environmental Working Group. Only three ingredients were actually listed by the manufacturer. Of those contaminants, one was linked to cancer and one was considered toxic to the brain and nervous system.

Inhaling Health Offenders

What kind of health effects could happen after sucking in air fresheners all day? Well, for starters, just simple allergies, such as a runny nose, watery eyes, coughing, and sneezing. Many people are allergic to artificial fragrances. If you think you have indoor allergies, perhaps you might want to simply remove air fresheners first and see if the problem improves. What's more, a study published in *New Scientist* found that women who live in a home with air fresheners are 25 percent more likely to have headaches.

The chemicals released into your indoor air by artificial fragrances can also aggravate asthma. Air fresheners contribute to poor indoor air quality, which is one of the leading asthma triggers. One study found that nearly one-third of people with asthma reported that they had breathing problems when exposed to air fresheners.

Then there are the long-term effects. There has not been adequate long-term testing of what health effects these myriad of chemicals have on your body after inhaling them all day. Ingredients used in artificial fragrances sometimes contain chemicals called phthalates. Phthalates are used as fragrance carriers, as well as being used in the formation of plastics. Some phthalates are thought to interrupt normal body development by mimicking the body's hormones of estrogen, testosterone, and thyroid hormones.

A More Natural Fragrance

There is nothing wrong with wanting a pleasantly scented home. There are times when air fresheners are actually warranted. Like when you are trying to hide the smells of a recipe gone wrong, or cover up the lingering effects of skunk smell that just doesn't seem to want to leave your dog. You will want to make sure that the ingredients of that fragrance, though, comes directly from the source, instead of a lab. For instance, why not just get the actual scent of a real-life rose or a pine tree, instead of an artificially created one?

Before switching fragrances, first eliminate the synthetic kinds. Get rid of any air fresheners in your home made with artificial fragrances, including plug-in units (with or without a night-light), stick units, sprays (including fabric fresheners), sneaker balls, hanging deodorizers in the closet or basement, trash can deodorizers (including scented trash can bags), as well as artificially fragranced diaper-pail deodorizers. Open the windows in your home and really air the place out for at least several hours, if not for a few days. Take care of the source of odors in your home.

QUESTION

What are essential oils?
Essential oils are highly concentrated aromatic essences that come directly from plants. The liquids are 75 to 100 times more concentrated than the oils found in dried herbs. Essential oils are often formed by extracting the aromatic properties of the plant from the leaves, flowers, bark, or other parts by steam distillation or cold pressing.

If you do like a fragrance in your home, choose products made entirely from essential oils. Beware of imitators that might say their product *contains* essential oils. It is common to use essential oils in combination with synthetic chemicals. Look for a product made only with 100 percent essential-oil fragrance. Aura Cacia (*www.auracacia.com*) has a great selection of home fragrances made solely from essential oils, such as sprays, diffusers, vaporizers, and lamp rings. Citrus Magic (*www.citrusmagic.com*) offers odor-eliminating sprays made from the peel of citrus fruits.

You can also make your own air freshener with essential oils. Simply pick a fragrance, or a combination thereof, and add eight to ten drops to a spray bottle of water. Spray throughout your home or wherever you need odor control. Keep in mind that essential oils are actually oil and might damage upholstery or fabrics, so do a patch test first. Other ways of naturally scenting your home are to simmer a pot of water with cinnamon sticks and cloves or vanilla, or use green cleaning products that are scented only with essential oils to leave a pleasant smell through your home.

Keeping Your Air Clean

Sure, there are plenty of ways that your indoor air can become contaminated. Every item that you use, from furniture to perfume, *will* be breathed in by you and your family. Do not kid yourself that these things are not finding a way inside your body. Thankfully, there are many ways that you can reduce that contamination and keep your indoor air healthy. Regardless of what method you choose, the simple fact is that you have just got to get more fresh air in and push the nasty air out.

Open Your Windows

Opening your windows and doors are the easiest and cheapest ways to ventilate your home. You just need to crack open the windows an inch or two or use a screen door to get air circulating. It is preferable to open windows or doors that are across from each other on opposite sides of the house. For example, open the window in your dining room and open the window in your living room, if they are located across from each other, to get a cross breeze and effectively push outdoor air through your home.

ALERT

Do not open your windows and doors during high allergen seasons if someone in your home is allergic to pollen. Also, do not open up your home to the outdoor air if your area is under a high smog advisory, or other type of health warning. You do not want to expose yourself to other health hazards unnecessarily.

Grow Fresh Air

When the folks at the National Aeronautics and Space Administration (NASA) decided to allow people to live in space on Skylab, they had to find a way to reduce the number of pollutants that accumulated in the indoor air. After all, astronauts can't just open the windows to get some fresh air circulation. Air pollution was a major concern, though, since 107 VOCs were detected in Skylab. What one scientist by the name of Dr. B.C. Wolverton found was that plants are actually wonderful air purifiers even in totally synthetic environments.

Houseplants are able to absorb the carbon dioxide that we give off and release oxygen in return. More surprising, though, is the fact that certain plants are especially well-suited at absorbing specific chemicals from the air, such as formaldehyde and benzene. In his book, *How to Grow Fresh Air*, Wolverton suggests fifty plants that have great VOC-absorbing qualities. Among them are:

- English ivy
- Golden pothos
- Gerber daisy
- Dracaena
- Snake plant
- Spider plant
- Philodendron
- Ferns
- Peace lily

There is not exact science as to how many plants you need inside your home for air purification. You certainly do not want to feel like you are living in a jungle. NASA studies have suggested that one houseplant for every 100 square feet of your home could effectively help purify your indoor air.

FACT

Kamal Meattle, a researcher who suffered from indoor air contamination, says that you need only three plants strategically placed in your house to purify the air: an areca palm to supply oxygen in your living room during the day, a mother-in-law's tongue to supply oxygen in the bedroom at night, and a money plant to remove VOCs.

Clean the House

A major part of keeping your indoor air quality healthy is to eliminate the particles in your home that can cause health problems. That means that you have got to vacuum and sweep regularly to eliminate dirt, dust, and other materials that get trapped in your flooring, which are re-released into the air every time someone walks across the floor. Dusting regularly is also important, too, in capturing and eliminating the nasty stuff that can fly through the air.

If you have pets, it is especially important to vacuum your floors and sweep as often as possible, even every day, to reduce the pet dander that can accumulate in your home. You also will want to vacuum or clean any furniture that your pet may lie on to eliminate pollution sources. Wash your pet's bedding frequently to reduce dust mites and pet dander.

Air Filtration Systems

Sometimes you might just not be able to use natural measures to purify your air. There are other ways that you can add an additional level of purification to your home's indoor air quality through mechanical means.

Ductwork Filters

You might already have an air filter that is built into your central heating and cooling system or furnace. These filters are typically square in shape and may have a flat or pleated filtering material inside that you can see. If your heating, ventilation, and air-conditioning system (HVAC) has an air filter of any kind, it is essential to clean or replace the filters regularly. If the filters are dirty and clogged with contaminants, they cannot effectively clean your air.

QUESTION

How often should I change my air filter?
A good rule of thumb is to change your disposable air filter with every change of the seasons, or roughly every three months. If you have heavy indoor contaminants, such as pet fur or smoke from a fireplace, it is wise to replace the filter more often, even every month or two.

All air filters for HVAC systems are not the same. Some will barely capture large particles, while others can capture very small pollutants. The difference is in the minimum efficiency reporting value (MERV) of an air filter. MERV ratings of an air filter range from one to twenty, with one being the lowest. Air filters with MERV values of one to four do not do much for your indoor air purification. These filters are essentially used to protect the HVAC system from particles that could damage it. For typical home use, look for filters with a MERV value of five to thirteen. These filters can remove smaller particles, especially filters with a MERV value between seven and thirteen which work very much like a High Efficiency Particulate Arresting (HEPA) filter. Higher MERV values, from fourteen to twenty, are unlikely to be found on filters that can be used in HVAC systems because the extremely high particle filtration would not work well with the system.

Room Air Filters

Stand-alone air purifiers that are designed to filter the air in one room can be highly effective at removing pollutants in spaces where you spend a lot of time. They are also great alternatives if you do not have a forced-air heating system in which you can install an air filter. When choosing an air purifier, you want a high number of CADR (the Clean Air Delivery Rate), based on how many cubic feet of air a purifier can filter a minute. Your air purifier should not generate ozone, though, as ozone can make lung problems and asthma worse. The Association of Home Appliance Manufacturer's Clean Air Delivery Rate website (*www.cadr.org*) allows you to compare and search for air purifiers based on CADR levels.

Many air purifiers use a HEPA filter that removes 99.7 percent of air pollutants .3 microns or larger from the air. To put that into perspective, pollen, mold, and other spores are .3 microns or larger, but bacteria and viruses are much smaller. The smaller the size of the micron that the air purifier can remove, the more pollutants there will be eliminated from your indoor air.

FACT

Ultra-low particulate air (ULPA) filters are the newest type of air filter on the market. ULPA filters have a serious degree of air filtration, removing 99.9995 percent of particles 0.12 microns or larger. The ability to remove so many particles, though, reduces the amount of air that can be cleaned with an ULPA filter.

Whole House Filters

Larger air filters, or air cleaners, that purify the air of your entire home are also available. These systems are much more costly and must be professionally installed. Whole-house air cleaners work with a forced-air heating system in which a large, box-shaped air filter is installed into the ductwork. They can be great at filtering your indoor air in every room of your home without much upkeep on your part, except for yearly filter changes.

CHECKLIST FOR HEALTHY INDOOR AIR

❏ Open your windows and doors to get fresh air in. This is the single most effective way to bring clean air into your home. Outdoor air is often much more healthy than indoor air, as long as there are not high-pollen or high-smog alerts.

❑ Dust, vacuum, and wash bedding frequently to kill dust mites. Dust mites are the source of many indoor allergies and asthma attacks. Killing the dust mites regularly will ensure that they cannot cause allergic reactions inside your home.

❑ Invest in the highest-quality air filters that you can. There will always be particles in the air that would be beneficial to remove, so invest in an air filter that can remove the greatest amount of particulates.

❑ Keep the humidity levels low in your home to control the growth of dust mites. Low humidity levels not only slow dust mite growth, but also can reduce mold growth.

❑ Make sure your heating systems work properly and have enough ventilation. Improperly installed heating and cooling systems can create poor indoor air quality problems that you might not be aware of.

❑ Eliminate synthetic air fresheners. Artificial fragrances are just a combination of synthetic chemicals being sprayed into your air for your family to inhale.

❑ Clean or replace your air filters regularly. Air filters cannot remove allergens and other particulates if they are clogged and not operating efficiently.

❑ Use essential oils for a healthy fragrance throughout your home. Plant-based fragrances come directly from nature and impart the actual scent of flowers, pine, etc.

❑ Add several houseplants to your home to naturally purify the air. Certain houseplants not only add beauty to your home, but can remove certain chemicals from the air naturally.

❑ Be aware of the synthetic ingredients that you bring into your home and how they can off-gas into your home's air. Our indoor air is polluted these days because of the excessive use of synthetic products, many of which release chemicals into your home for months and years.

CHAPTER 4

Water Quality

You drink it, you cook with it, you bathe in it, you wash your dishes with it. Your home's water is an integral part to every aspect of your daily life. If your water contains questionable materials, though, you might unknowingly be exposing yourself and your family to toxic chemicals with every sip you take. Your water could be totally safe. Or your water could contain substances like lead. The only way to know for sure is to take matters in your own hands and find out for yourself.

Safe Drinking Water Act

You probably always have relatively safe drinking water coming out of your tap on demand any time you want. Be thankful, because millions of people around the world do not. However, there is always room for improvement in the quality of water that comes out in American homes.

Who Is Affected?

The Safe Drinking Water Act (SDWA) was passed by Congress in 1974 to protect Americans' public drinking water supply. This act, which was most recently amended in 1996, is the main federal law that ensures you have safe drinking water coming out of your tap. Under the SDWA, the EPA decides the federal limits of contaminants allowed in your water and oversees the entities responsible for supplying the public water.

ALERT

Approximately 15 percent of Americans get drinking water from their own wells. The SDWA does not regulate the water quality coming from private wells that serve fewer than twenty-five people. The EPA has a website (*http://water.epa.gov/drink/info/well/index.cfm*) with specific information on how to keep private drinking water wells safe.

The SDWA oversees the water for the majority of Americans. Any public drinking water system, whether private or public, that serves at least twenty-five people or fifteen service connections for at least sixty days a year falls under the SDWA. The United States has approximately 155,00 public water systems.

Consumer's Right to Know

As part of the SDWA, approximately 53,000 community water systems (CWS) across America are required to provide an annual consumer confidence report (often called a drinking-water quality report). A CWS is a public water supplier that serves the same people daily throughout the year. More than 273 million people are served by a CWS each year. If you are served by a CWS, you should receive a consumer confidence report by July 1 of each year. You might get the report in your water bill or as a separate mailing. Smaller water systems that serve less than 10,000 people can publish the information in another way, such as posting it in the local newspaper. In the consumer confidence report, you can find a list of regulated contaminants that were detected in the treated water by your CWS and the levels of those contaminants from the preceding year.

Any community water system that serves more than 100,000 people must post its consumer confidence report online for public access. Smaller water suppliers might also post their reports online, though they are not required. The EPA has a search engine (*http://cfpub.epa.gov/safewater/ccr/index.cfm*) that helps you find your drinking water supplier by state and links to their annual online drinking water quality report if available.

Drinking Water Contaminants

The EPA currently regulates more than ninety different contaminants in drinking water and sets maximum allowable levels through the SDWA. The entire list can be found on the EPA's Drinking Water Contaminants website (*http://water.epa.gov/drink/contaminants/index.cfm*). There are many, many more than ninety contaminants that can enter your water, though. According to an Environmental Working Group analysis, there were 315 pollutants found in drinking water across the United States between 2004 and 2009. A multitude of sources, such as mining and industrial waste, can add chemicals to waterways that the EPA has not set limits for and for which the health risks are not even known yet. It is wise to remove as many contaminants from your water as possible, but there are several documented high-risk contaminants that cause the most concern.

ALERT

Perchlorate is the newest contaminant to be regulated under the SDWA. The chemical is used to produce rocket fuels, fireworks, and explosives and has been found in the nation's water supply. Perchlorate is linked to disruption of the thyroid. The EPA has not yet set the legal limit for perchlorate, therefore your public water system might not test for the substance.

Lead

Lead is regulated by the SDWA for maximum allowable levels in your drinking water. Yet many people ingest more lead than is legally allowed every time they turn on their tap. In fact, the EPA estimates that up to 20 percent of your lead exposure may come from lead in your drinking water. How is that possible? The problem lies within a home's plumbing system.

Lead can enter your drinking water if your plumbing materials contain lead. When the plumbing materials start to corrode, the lead can then be released into your water as it travels through the pipes. It is not just older homes that have a lead plumbing problem, though. Even newer homes made with "lead-free" plumbing can have lead corrosion problems. After August 6, 1998, it became illegal to sell any pipe or plumbing fitting or fixture that is not lead-free for use in homes. However, it is still legal to have as much as 8 percent lead content in plumbing labeled "lead-free." Other factors can also influence how much lead leaches into your drinking water, including the types and amounts of minerals in your water, as well as the acidity of the water.

FACT

The new "Reduction of Lead in Drinking Water Act" will reduce the amount of lead that can be contained in faucets, fittings, and valves from 8 percent to 0.25 percent beginning in January 2014. Two states are not waiting that long for regulation, though. California and Vermont already have laws mandating the lower lead limit in their states.

There is great concern about lead being in your drinking water because the metal can cause some major health problems. Even short-term exposure to lead can cause negative health problems. Lead is thought to contribute to mental developmental delays, shortened attention spans, blood pressure increases, hearing and learning disabilities, stroke, kidney disease, and cancer.

To help prevent additional lead exposure through your tap water, you should flush out your pipes any time that the water has not been used for more than six hours. That means to let your cold water run as long as it takes until the water gets as cold as it will get. It might take several seconds, but it could also take as long as two minutes. This flushing action allows any water that has been sitting in lead-containing pipes that might have absorbed higher amounts of lead to be pushed through your plumbing fixtures and allow fresh water to be delivered in its place. When using tap water for cooking and drinking, choose cold water instead of hot water, because hot water can make lead dissolve more rapidly from lead-containing pipes.

Bacteria, Viruses, and Parasites

Bacteria, viruses, and parasites are all considered pathogens, which can cause disease. While there is much concern about spreading bacteria and viruses through the air or by direct contact, it is also possible to be exposed through your water. Chlorine and other disinfectants are added to drinking water to kill those pathogens.

FACT

You can kill pathogens in your drinking water by boiling the water at a full boil for at least one minute. Higher altitudes require a longer boiling time. This is an effective way to kill pathogens if you do not want to use a filter created especially to remove pathogens.

The SDWA regulates certain pathogens in drinking water. *Cryptosporidium*, a parasite that is common if water is contaminated with sewage or animal waste, is regulated because it can cause diarrhea, vomiting, and cramps. *Giardia lamblia* is another parasite that can also cause nausea, headaches, and cramps. It is also found in water contaminated with human or animal waste. *Legionella* bacteria and many viruses are regulated due to their health risks, as well. People with compromised immune systems must be careful about their exposure to even the legal limits of these pathogens allowed in drinking water and often need to filter their water specifically to remove these pathogens.

Chlorine

Chlorine is among the most recognizable contaminants because you can smell and taste the chemical in your water. Chlorine is added to kill pathogens, but even with the positive health benefits of killing pathogens, there is still a legal limit of how much chlorine can be present in your water. Eye and nose irritation, as well as stomach discomfort, are the health risks of ingesting chlorine in drinking water. Byproducts from adding chlorine to the water may pose health hazards, too, though research is still being done.

Fluoride

Fluoride might not necessarily be considered a contaminant, since many water utilities purposely add fluoride to the drinking water. There is much debate on the health effects of fluoride in drinking water, though, and many people would like to limit their exposure to the mineral.

In the 1930s, researchers found that people had fewer cavities if they consumed naturally fluoridated water while they were young. Some areas have drinking water where natural fluoride levels are high, but not all areas do, so fluoride started being added to some water systems to help protect people against cavities. The EPA does not require the addition of fluoride in drinking water. It is a decision that local water systems make as to whether or not to add fluoride into the water.

The levels of acceptable fluoride in your drinking water can be confusing. The EPA currently has a maximum allowable limit of 4.0 parts per million. However, the EPA also has a secondary limit for fluoride set at 2.0 ppm. The EPA cannot enforce the secondary limit, though it suggests the limit for cosmetic health effects, such as tooth discoloration. Some government agencies advise an ever lower limit, though. The CDC and U.S. Public Health Service suggest fluoride levels in water should be between 0.7 and 1.2 ppm. The EPA is re-evaluating its maximum limits of fluoride that are allowed in public drinking water. With so many differing levels of fluoride that are suggested or actually enforced, you should find out how much fluoride, if any, is actually in your drinking water and compare it to the levels suggested for both health and cosmetic safety.

ESSENTIAL

To find out whether your drinking water has fluoride added, you can read your water system's consumer confidence report or visit the My Water's Fluoride website run by the Centers for Disease Control and Prevention (*http://apps.nccd.cdc.gov/MWF/Index.asp*). Only thirty-nine states participate in the website, though, so you may need to ask your water supplier directly about the addition of fluoride in your drinking water.

Excessive use of fluoride has been linked to bone fractures and pain and tenderness in the bones of adults, as well as pitting of tooth enamel in children. To reduce your exposure to fluoride, evaluate your dental care products, including toothpaste and mouthwashes, to see if fluoride is added. For young children, the primary source of fluoride exposure is swallowing fluoridated toothpaste, so use only a small amount, such as the size of a pea. Talk with your dentist about your concerns of too much fluoride.

Testing Your Water

If you receive a consumer confidence report from your drinking water supplier, then you have a good understanding of what contaminants were found in your water in the previous year. The report will tell you what contaminants were found, the levels of those contaminants, and how the levels compare to the EPA's maximum contaminant level. But even people who receive a consumer confidence report might still want additional testing done.

Who Should Test Their Water

Everyone should test his or her water for lead, because lead exposure is often a problem within a home, and not from the water source. The only way to know if there is lead in your drinking water is to test it.

If your drinking water is from a private well, you should definitely test your water. If you are concerned about other chemicals that might be in your water that are not regulated by the EPA, you should have a private laboratory test your water. If you live in an agricultural area where there is a high amount of pesticide use, you should have your water tested for pesticides residues, many of which are not regulated by the EPA. Likewise, if you live in an area close to a waste dump or other site with heavy pollution, you should have your water tested for a broad range of chemicals that might be contaminating your water that your water utilities are not required by law to test for.

How to Test Your Water

You will want to find a reputable laboratory that can efficiently test your drinking water and provide you with accurate results. The EPA lists the certifying officers for drinking water in each state (*http://water.epa.gov/scitech/drinkingwater/labcert/statecertification.cfm*) with links to their websites. On each site you can find the certified laboratories that can perform drinking water tests in your state. You can also test your water through private-sector laboratories such as National Testing Laboratories Ltd. (*www.watercheck.com*) and Suburban Water Testing Labs (*www.h2otest.com*). Contact your local health department to see if they offer lead tests for your drinking water or tests for other contaminants.

Filtering Your Tap Water

Maybe you want to filter your tap water because you do not like the taste. Perhaps you have found a contaminant in your drinking water that you want removed. Or you just want to play it safe and filter as many contaminants out of your drinking water as possible, regardless of what the tests might say. Adding a filter to your home's water supply is a smart choice that allows you to be in more control of what ends up in your drinking water. With more than 40 percent of Americans investing in a water filter, it seems that many people are concerned about the quality of their tap water.

Not all water filters are the same, though. Some are more effective at removing certain contaminants than others. The following are some common contaminants and what kind of filter it takes to remove them from your water, according to the EPA:

Water Contaminant	Filter Needed to Remove Contaminant
Lead	Distillation, reverse osmosis, and some carbon filters
Giardia and *Cryptosporidum*	Distillation, reverse osmosis, ultraviolet light, absolute one-micron filters, and filters certified for cyst removal
Nitrates	Distillation, reverse osmosis, and ion exchange
Pesticides	Some carbon filters
Radon	Activated carbon filter and aeration
Bacteria and viruses	Distillation, reverse osmosis, ultraviolet light, and disinfection

If you are concerned about removing a particular contaminant, be sure to purchase a filter that has been proven to remove that contaminant. If you want to clean up your drinking water as much as possible, you will want a system that combines different types of filtering agents to remove many contaminants. Look for water filter manufacturers that can supply you with research of how much of each contaminant is removed with the filter. This information is often available on the package or on the company's website. You can then compare the percentages of contaminants removed and pick the one that you think would work best for your situation.

Pitcher and Faucet Filters

One of the easiest ways to filter tap water is to purchase a pitcher with a water filter built in. You simply fill the pitcher with normal tap water and the carbon filter will draw out impurities as the water settles into the pitcher. These types of filters are less expensive at first, but the filter often has to be changed frequently, which can increase the cost. Most pitcher filters use a carbon-based filter, which are good at improving the taste of your water as well as filtering out some contaminants. These types of filters will generally not remove as many contaminants as other types of filters, so be sure to read the labels and determine what the filter will actually remove.

Other types of faucet filters can be a system that is easily attached to your plumbing and sits on the counter or can be hidden under the sink. These types of filters can allow you to switch between using normal tap water, such as for doing dishes, and filtered tap water that you use for cooking and drinking. Countertop and under-the-sink models generally have an additional faucet that you install to dispense filtered water.

ALERT

It can be really easy to forget when you installed a new filter in your water pitcher or faucet filter. Write the date down on a sticker that you can attach to the system. You can also figure out the time frame when you will need to purchase a new filter and add it to your calendar as a reminder.

Filters attached to the faucet directly might need to have the filter changed more frequently, but countertop and under-the-sink models generally only need a filter change once or twice a year. Pur (*www.purwater .com*) and Brita (*www.brita.com*) make pitcher filters and faucet-mounted water filters. Aquasana (*www.aquasana.com*), Paragon Water Systems (*www.paragonwater.com*), and Multi-Pure Drinking Water Systems (*www .multipureco.com*) offer countertop and under-the-sink models.

Distillation

Distillation water filters can be placed on your countertop to filter water, but they can be slow and more costly. Distillation heats water to its boiling point, which kills microbes. The pure water vapor rises, leaving the contaminants behind. The water vapor then condenses and accumulates in an attached pitcher for you to drink. Distilled water might have a distinct taste, because the natural minerals of the water have been removed. Waterwise (*www.waterwise.com*) makes a wide range of water distillers.

Reverse Osmosis

Reverse-osmosis systems are costly, but they are highly effective. A reverse-osmosis water filter forces water through a membrane that absorbs many contaminants in the water. This type of water filter is extremely effective at reducing most chemical contaminants and eliminating disease-causing organisms, such as bacteria, viruses, *Giardia,* and *Cryptosporidium.* Many reverse-osmosis systems actually waste three to four gallons of water for every gallon of water that they purify. More efficient models are available, so be sure to look for them when choosing a filter. Watts Premier (*www.watts premier.com*) and Multi-Pure Drinking Water Systems (*www.multipureco.com*) are among the manufacturers with reverse-osmosis water filtration systems.

Whole House Filters

You can eliminate the need to fill pitchers or remember to use a special faucet if you use a whole home water filter. These expensive filters must be installed by a plumber. The system will filter out impurities such as chlorine from every single tap in your house, including water in the bathroom for bathing and brushing your teeth, as well as cooking and drinking water in the kitchen. While chlorine is primarily the contaminant that is removed from these systems, check to see what other contaminants might also be eliminated in particular filters. Watts Premier (*www.wattspremier.com*) and Aquasana (*www.aquasana.com*) make whole house filter systems.

Bottled Water

Many people purchase bottled water because they are concerned about drinking tap water. Bottled water is somehow thought to be purer and healthier than what is coming out of the tap. Ironically, this is not the case. In fact, you might be spending more money for water that is actually less healthy than what you can get for free.

Different Regulations

Bottled water and tap water are regulated by two different agencies in two different ways. Tap water is regulated by the EPA. Bottled water, though, is regulated by the U.S. Food and Drug Administration (FDA), and is actually considered a food for regulation purposes. The FDA does not do its own health and safety testing. It relies on the manufacturers of the product to do that. While the FDA has legal standards on the books for health and safety that manufacturers are supposed to follow by law, it might only be notified about possible health hazards in a product after an inspection at a plant. However, according to the FDA, "bottled water plants generally are assigned a relatively low priority for inspection."

All public water systems must publish water quality tests each year identifying what is in the tap water. Bottled water companies are not required by federal law to give the public any information about what is in the bottled water. Since FDA inspections do not occur frequently, and water quality reports of bottled water are often not published for public inspection, there is cause for concern about finding out what exactly is in your bottled water.

FACT

A California law that went into effect in 2009 requires bottled water companies to label the name and location of their water source and provide consumers with water quality testing reports, which includes the treatment process, on request. This law applies only to bottled water sold within the state of California.

Marketing Claims

If you read any bottled water label, you will likely be led to believe that the water quality far exceeds anything that could come out of your tap. Many labels tout the claims that the water is "pure," "natural spring water," or filtered by the earth to naturally remove any impurities. There are no laws regarding these marketing claims, and the water source might be the exact same source that supplies your tap water. The Environmental Working Group (EWG) found thirty-eight pollutants in ten bottled water brands that they tested in 2008. Two of those bottled water brands actually had pollutant levels that exceeded state and industry health standards.

ESSENTIAL

Find out what is in your favorite bottled water at *www.ewg.org/ health/report/BottledWater/Bottled-Water-Scorecard/Search*. This handy website lists bottled waters by brand name, and you can click on each brand to see the source of the water, the purification methods, what testing has been done, and the water quality report.

The EPA states that "Bottled water is not necessarily safer than your tap water." The agency also says that "Some bottled water is treated more than tap water, while some is treated less or not treated at all," and adds that "Consumers who choose to purchase bottled water should carefully read its label to understand what they are buying, whether it is a better taste, or a certain method of treatment." If you are buying bottled water because you believe that it is healthier, you must do all of the research on your own to find out how your bottled water has been treated, what contaminants might be in the water, and whether it is any safer than what you can get for free out of your kitchen sink.

CHECKLIST FOR HEALTHY WATER

❑ Find out what it is in your drinking water by looking at your consumer confidence report or asking your water system for a water quality report. The only way to know what is lurking in your drinking water is to read your water quality report. It will tell you exactly which chemicals and minerals are in the water and at what concentrations.

❑ If you have a private well, have your water tested. If you have a private well, it is imperative for you to test your water because no one else is monitoring its safety. Pollutants change throughout the years, and just because it was safe many years ago, does not mean that it still is.

❑ Allow your tap water to run until cold before drinking it. This method ensures that standing water has been flushed through the pipes and does not contain lead from sitting in the pipes for too long.

❑ Have your tap water tested for lead. Even though a water quality report does not show lead in your water, it could still be there at high concentrations if your indoor plumbing contains lead.

❑ Determine whether fluoride is added to your drinking water, and how much you are getting throughout the day. There are many different schools of thought about having fluoride in your water, so find out at which concentration fluoride might be in your water and what effects it could have.

❑ Boil your water if you are concerned about pathogens. High heat will kill bacteria in your drinking water, but will not remove chemicals.

❏ Allow chlorine to evaporate naturally in a pitcher if you are not using a filter. Chlorine can naturally release out of water if left uncovered for a day or so.

❏ Invest in a water filter to remove contaminants and improve the taste of your tap water. Though water treatment plants should be removing pollutants, you can remove even more of the ones that you are concerned about with personal water filters.

❏ Avoid bottled water when possible. Surprisingly, bottled water is less regulated than tap water, which means you could be putting yourself at more risk to contaminants.

❏ Investigate the health standards and safety tests of the bottled water manufacturers that you purchase. With little regulation, you should be very concerned about the source and bottling methods of the bottled water that you choose.

CHAPTER 5

EMFs and Radiation

If you have ever tried functioning normally in your home during a power outage, you know that many of the things that you use every day run on electricity. Electrical and wireless devices make our lives easier, but they might also affect your health. There is no need to give up the wonders of modern-day conveniences and revert back to the Dark Ages, though, as long as you use some simple precautions to protect yourself and your family throughout the day.

Radiation

Radiation can be found everywhere. Surprising, but true. When most people talk about radiation exposure, they might think of nuclear power plant leaks, X-rays at the doctor's office, or airport security screening measures. But just stepping outside will expose you to radiation from the sun. Whether natural or man-made, understanding where radiation comes from can help you reduce your exposure.

ESSENTIAL

A round-trip flight from New York City to Los Angeles will expose you to half of the amount of radiation that you would receive from one chest X-ray. The radiation exposure comes from cosmic radiation in the atmosphere, and at high altitudes, your exposure is much higher than on the ground.

Different Types of Radiation

Radiation is the energy that is emitted from any source. It does not have to be man-made energy. It can be as simple as the heat and light coming off of the sun every day, too. Different sources have different amounts of radiation. The following are the main sources of radiation, from the highest amount of radiation exposure to the lowest:

- Gamma rays
- X-rays
- Ultraviolet (UV) rays
- Visible light
- Infrared rays
- Microwaves
- Radiofrequency (radio) waves
- Extremely low-frequency (ELF) radiation

Though all radiation is energy, there are two different types of radiation, ionizing and non-ionizing. The difference between the two is how a molecule is affected by the radiation. Non-ionizing radiation is what you are typically exposed to each day. It is a low-frequency radiation that can move around the parts of a molecule and cause them to vibrate, but does not alter the molecule. Since the molecules are not damaged, non-ionizing radiation is not known to increase your cancer risk.

Ionizing radiation is much more dangerous because it can permanently change a molecule. Ionizing radiation can cause electrons to be removed from an atom, which creates an ion. When that happens, there is the original molecule that has been altered, and an additional ion molecule that has an electric charge. This process can damage your cells, which increases your cancer risk.

Where the Radiation Comes From

There are many different uses for non-ionizing radiation, and you will encounter them each day. Power lines create non-ionizing radiation. The radio waves coming from your favorite radio station are a form of non-ionizing radiation. Those heat lamps that keep your food warm at a restaurant use non-ionizing radiation, as do microwave ovens.

Ionizing radiation can come from both natural and unnatural sources. The natural sources of radiation are lumped together and called background radiation. This radiation comes from naturally occurring radioactive materials in the environment, such as rocks and radon, as well as cosmic radiation coming from outer space. Radon is the biggest source of ionizing radiation, accounting for more than half of the average American's radiation exposure each year. Ionizing radiation can also come from man-made sources, such as tanning booths, medical X-rays, and diagnostic procedures that use nuclear medicine. Nuclear power plants and nuclear weapons testing can also be a source of ionizing radiation.

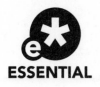

ESSENTIAL

People who live at higher elevations receive increased exposure to radiation. Cosmic radiation from outer space affects us here on earth, but the farther you are from the source, the less radiation you will be exposed to. That is why residents of Utah, with higher elevations, will be exposed to more cosmic radiation than residents of Florida, who live near sea level.

Wondering just how much radiation you might be exposed to on a daily basis? You can calculate your radiation dose with the EPA's radiation calculator (*www.epa.gov/radiation/understand/calculate.html*). By inputting lifestyle habits such as where you live, how much you travel, and your television and computer usage, you can get an estimate of how much radiation you are exposed to each year.

Radiation and Increased Cancer Risk

Due to the nature of ionizing radiation, it already has been proven that ionizing radiation can be harmful to your health. In fact, ionizing radiation is a proven human carcinogen. Ionizing radiation alters molecules, which means that it can damage cells in your body. Your body can repair the damage, but sometimes things might not go quite right. Perhaps the damage is too great to be repaired or the process of repairing damaged cells might not go as it should, leading to cancerous cells.

ALERT

Smoking, which increases your cancer risk, can also be a source of radiation. Tobacco traps naturally occurring radioactive minerals on its sticky leaves. When the tobacco is processed into cigarettes, the radioactive minerals are not removed. Cigarette smokers then inhale those radioactive minerals while smoking. Secondhand smoke can contain the same radioactive materials, as well.

Cancer is definitely a health risk associated with long-term exposure to ionizing radiation. Leukemia is the most common radiation-induced cancer. While any cancer can develop from radiation exposure, some of the other cancers most strongly related to radiation exposure are:

- Lung cancer
- Skin cancer
- Thyroid cancer
- Multiple myeloma
- Breast cancer
- Stomach cancer

Radiation exposure can also cause mutations. Some mutations are in a specific individual, such as an infant born with a birth defect because of exposure to radiation. Other mutations alter the genes of an individual and become genetic mutations, which are inherited and passed down through generations.

Research is still being done on potential health risks from non-ionizing radiation, though it is not known to increase cancer risk. That is good news since the majority of radiation that individuals receive each year is non-ionizing radiation, not the damaging ionizing radiation. However, limiting the cumulative doses of all radiation that you receive each and every day could protect your health.

What Is an EMF?

Electric and magnetic fields, known as EMFs, are non-ionizing sources of radiation. EMFs are areas of energy that surround electrical devices that are plugged in and turned on. You cannot see them or feel them, but EMFs exist around anything that runs on electricity in your house. Not only do EMFs exist around the appliances and devices that you plug into an electric socket, but EMFs exist around the electric wiring and panels that help supply electricity to your house, too.

Where EMFs Come From

While EMFs are generated around anything that uses or transports electricity, the amount of EMFs that you are exposed to will vary depending on how close you are to the source. EMFs disappear rapidly with distance, so the farther that you position yourself from an appliance, the less exposure you will receive. For instance, if you stand right next to a microwave oven, your EMF exposure will be higher than if you stand three feet away.

The same is true for EMF exposure from power lines outside of your home. Not all power lines are the same. Some have much larger EMF exposures than others. Power lines that must send large amounts of electricity from the generating plants to cities are likely to have larger EMF exposures than the power lines that run on a suburban street, though there are many factors that affect the EMF levels. Regardless of which type of power line it is, the farther that you are from the lines, the less exposure you will have. The Connecticut Department of Public Health states that at 300 feet, about the length of a football field, the EMF levels from power lines would be considered "background levels," which means that the EMF exposure is similar to what is commonly found and not unusually higher.

EMFs are not blocked by walls. Just because you are in a house does not mean that you would be protected from increased levels of EMF exposure located outside your home. Inside your house, if one room contains excessive EMF levels, the walls of your home will not block those EMFs from traveling into other rooms.

Measuring EMF Levels

You can find out just how many EMFs you and your family are exposed to at home with a simple electronic gadget known as a gaussmeter. EMFs are measured in units called gauss (G). Measurements in the home will most often be calculated by milligauss (mG), which is 1,000 times smaller than a gauss. A gaussmeter can measure the EMF that exists in any room or around any specific electrical device.

FACT

Gaussmeters aren't just for homeowners trying to reduce their radiation exposure. They are also widely used by ghost-hunters, too. It is thought that spikes in EMF levels, compared to a normal baseline level with no other logical explanation, indicates the presence of a ghost manifesting itself.

Gaussmeters can be purchased online and at some home improvement stores. You can also ask your electric company or electric cooperative if they can do an EMF assessment of your home. Some companies will perform the service for free or for a small charge.

Unknown Health Effects of EMFs

In the 1980s, some studies suggested that there was a link between EMF exposure and childhood leukemia. But after two decades of research by the National Institute of Health's National Institute of Environmental Health Sciences (NIEHS), no definitive connection could be found between EMF exposures and childhood leukemia.

Though the NIEHS could not prove an undisputed link between EMF exposure and childhood leukemia, they have stated that "the overall pattern of results suggests a weak association between increasing exposure to EMFs and an increased risk of childhood leukemia."

While there are no definite answers whether EMF exposures can cause health problems, many people just do not want to take the risk if it is not necessary. In fact, even though the NIEHS could not find any direct links, they still recommend "practical ways of reducing exposures to EMFs."

EMF Sources in the Home

Though you can be exposed to EMF anywhere, your home might be a major source of EMF levels. With all of the gadgets and devices that can be plugged in at home throughout the day, you might have EMF hot spots that you are not even aware of. The good news is that you can control your exposure to EMF levels inside your home by simply moving some things around or unplugging some appliances when not in use.

Televisions and Computers

Do you sit in front of a computer all day at work? Then do you come home and relax by watching a few hours of TV? You could unknowingly be exposing yourself to very low levels of radiation with every hour you spend in front of a computer or television.

Some television and computer monitors use a cathode ray tube, which can create low levels of X-rays. Keep in mind that X-rays contain ionizing radiation, the kind that can cause health problems. Flat screen televisions and computer monitors that have a plasma display or Liquid Crystal Display (LCD) do not use cathode ray tubes, which means that they do not produce X-rays. As electronic devices, all computers and televisions, not just ones with a tube display, will radiate EMFs, as well.

There have been no medical links between TV or computer monitor X-ray emissions and health problems. The FDA limits the amount of radiation that can be emitted from a TV to 0.5 milliroentgen (mR) per hour. Even so, you might still want to limit your radiation exposure that comes from a television or computer using a cathode ray tube.

As with all radiation sources, the farther you are from the device creating the radiation, the less exposure you will have. If you have a TV or computer that uses a cathode ray tube, sit as far away as possible (at least two to three feet) to reduce your exposure. Limit your time spent on the computer or watching TV. When it comes time to purchase a new television or computer monitor, choose an LCD or plasma screen.

Home Electronics

Other electronic devices in your home can emit EMFs and radiation. When these devices are turned off or unplugged, they cannot emit radiation. While all electronic devices will have an EMF field, some devices are more worrisome than others.

Electric blankets can emit a magnetic field that lies right on top of your body. Do not sleep with an electric blanket plugged in. If you want to warm your bed before sleeping, turn on the electric blanket before getting into bed, and make sure to turn it off and unplug it before sleeping. Water bed heaters will also emit EMFs.

Electric clocks have a surprisingly high EMF exposure, considering how small they are. Unfortunately, most people have an electric clock right on their bedside table, close to their head while sleeping. Position electric clocks so they are at least six feet from you, especially when you are lying in bed. Even better, choose battery-operated or windup clocks to reduce your EMF exposure.

Hair dryers are another common electronic device with a surprisingly high EMF exposure. Since hair dryers are aimed directly at the head, there is concern about increased EMF exposure. Low-EMF hair dryers are available. You can also let your hair completely air-dry when possible, or allow your hair to dry as long as possible before styling with a hair dryer.

Electrical Sources and Wiring

Appliances and other items that run off of electricity are not the only sources of EMF exposure in your home. The places where electricity comes into your home can be a high source of EMF exposure, too. If you know where EMFs are elevated in your home, you can avoid them or fix them.

Certain parts of your home might have higher-than-average EMF levels that you cannot easily change. For instance, the spot where your electricity meter is connected to your home, especially if it is an old, rotating disc meter, could have higher-than-average EMF levels. Other electricity connections, such as the main distribution panels, fuse boxes, backup power supplies, and places with major wiring, might also register high levels of EMFs.

Knowing where these areas are in your home allows you to arrange your daily routine so that you do not stay in a high-EMF area of your home for too long. For instance, you do not want to put a bed where you sleep for eight to nine hours a night against a wall with a high EMF reading if you can move the bed to another location. If your fuse box is located in a bedroom of the house, you might not want to make that room a nursery for a newborn child.

ALERT

Since EMFs are not blocked by walls, it does not matter if an electrical source with a high EMF reading is physically located within a room or not. Your family can still be exposed to the EMFs because the waves will travel to adjacent areas. However, the EMFs will diminish in strength the farther away that you get.

If the wiring in your home is faulty in any way, it can also cause an increased EMF exposure to you and your family. Electrical wires that have been installed properly should not have elevated EMF levels. However, if the wiring was not installed properly, or if a problem has started with your home's wiring, EMF levels can start rising unnecessarily. The only way to know for sure whether faulty wiring is causing high EMF levels is to test your home with a gaussmeter.

Microwaves

Microwave ovens use non-ionizing radiation to heat food. The radiation causes the water molecules in the food to vibrate, which in turn produces heat and makes the food cook faster. There are regulations for the amount of radiation that a microwave can emit during operation. If the microwave is not operated according to instructions, though, or is damaged in any way, excessive amounts of microwave radiation can escape, especially if a microwave door does not close properly. If your microwave door is bent or cracked, if the door seal is not tight because it is dirty, or if the door does not close properly after excessive use, you might be exposed to higher levels of microwave radiation than the FDA has allowed. Check your microwave to make sure that it is operating properly, and never lean directly against a microwave while it is heating food.

FACT

Microwaves cause water, fat, and sugar molecules to vibrate 2.5 million times per second. The vibration causes heat, but takes a while to stop. That is why instructions often say to let the food sit for a minute or two after cooking. As the molecules slow down, the food will still continue to cook even after the microwave is off.

Microwaves do not make food radioactive. The waves used in microwave cooking are similar to television and radio waves. Microwaves only penetrate food to a depth of one to one and half inches and cause vibrations that heat the food to the inner core.

Cell Phones

Though it might seem that cell phones have always been around, they are actually still quite new in the relative scheme of things. Cell phones did not become popular until the 1990s, and wireless technology has been rapidly growing in leaps and bounds over the past two decades. Medical research is still trying to catch up with this new way of living and determine whether or not wireless technology could have any damaging health effects.

Wireless technology, including cell phones, uses radio frequency (RF), which is a non-ionizing form of radiation. Even though the non-ionizing form of radiation is not supposed to be a health risk, there is evidence that cell phone radiation can cause cancer. The World Health Organization has said that personal cell phone use is "possibly carcinogenic to humans," although further studies are still being done.

Is that a reason to ditch your cell phone? Probably not, but there are certain ways you can use your mobile phone that will reduce your risk. Do not use your cell phone for lengthy conversations if a conventional, wired phone is available. Use a hands-free device when talking on your cell phone to reduce the RF waves being emitted close to your head.

You might even want to change your cell phone. Different types of cell phones have different specific absorption rates (SAR). The SAR is the amount of RF energy that is absorbed from the phone into a person's body. While all cell phones are different, manufacturers are required to report the SAR values of their phones to the Federal Communications Commission (FCC). Sometimes the SAR level is located inside the battery compartment of your phone. If the level is not listed on the phone, you can find the phone's FCC ID number, usually located somewhere on the phone, such as under the battery pack, and try searching the FCC database (*http://transition.fcc.gov/oet/ea/fccid/*) to find the SAR level. Lower SAR levels are preferable to higher SAR levels, though the highest legal amount is 1.6 watts per kilogram (W/kg).

Sunlight

The sun that shines upon you every day is a sometimes-confusing source of radiation. Is it ionizing radiation? Is it non-ionizing radiation? The answer, it seems, is a little bit of both. Sunlight is made of ultraviolet (UV) radiation. UV rays fall in the middle of the spectrum of ionizing and non-ionizing radiation. They are not as powerful as X-rays, but they have more energy, and therefore more radiation, than visible light.

You probably know that sunlight can cause skin cancer. That is why UV rays are similar to ionizing radiation. But UV rays can only penetrate so far into your body, so they would not affect other organ systems other than skin. UV rays can also have different radiation exposures. UVA rays are the weakest of the UV rays and, while they might lead to cancer, their main health hazard is premature skin damage such as wrinkles. UVB rays are a little stronger than UVA and can cause damage to DNA, which means that they can cause skin cancer. Sunscreens can actually prevent UV radiation from reaching the skin, creating a chemical barrier on your skin's surface. The higher the SPF protection that a sunscreen offers, the more UVB rays will be blocked. For instance, according to the Skin Cancer Foundation, an SPF 15 will block about 93 percent of UVB rays, while SPF 50 blocks about 98 percent. For the greatest protection from UV rays, use a broad spectrum sunscreen, with both UVA and UVB protection, and reapply at least every two hours.

CHECKLIST TO REDUCE YOUR RADIATION AND EMF EXPOSURE

❑ Do not position a bed against a wall with an electrical source such as a fuse box or electric meter. Extremely high levels of EMF could be surrounding electrical sources, and they are not blocked by walls. Do not position furniture that you spend a lot of time on, such as a bed, near these EMF hot spots.

❑ Do not spend excessive time in areas of your home with high EMF levels that you cannot fix. EMF levels can be higher in certain parts of your home, but you might not be able to fix those problems. To reduce your exposure, do not spend the greatest majority of your time in those areas.

❑ Check your microwave door to ensure that it seals properly. Improperly working microwaves can emit high amounts of radiation through cracks and openings.

❑ Move a bedside clock as far away as possible, or switch to a nonelectronic version. Electric clocks can emit high EMFs, and most clocks are positioned right next to your head on a bedside table while you are sleeping.

❑ Limit excessive use of cell phones and use a hands-free device. By reducing the amount of time that a cell phone is placed against your ear and skull, you reduce your exposure to nonionizing radiation.

❑ Move your computer monitor to at least an arm's length away from your body, and your television to at least two to three feet away. All electronics emit EMFs, and old CRT screens and monitors can emit X-rays while operating.

❏ Turn off electrical devices when not in use, if possible. Turning off the power to an electrical device often can eliminate the EMFs that it is emitting.

❏ Limit your use of hair dryers or invest in a low-EMF model. Hair dryers can have high EMF fields beside your head, so let your hair air-dry as much as possible before using a hair dryer.

❏ Check your cell phone's SAR level. Some phones emit higher energy levels than others, but all cell phone manufacturers are required to report their levels to the FCC.

❏ Protect yourself from the sun's UV rays. The sun emits radiation, so protect yourself by limiting time in the sun and using sunscreens.

CHAPTER 6

Decorating Your Home

The furniture and décor that you decorate your home with makes a statement about you—your personality, your tastes, and your family. You don't have to change your sense of style, but there are some suggestions that you want to keep in mind when shopping for items for your home. Choosing nontoxic décor that will grace your home for years to come is healthy for your family and a sign of great taste.

Furniture—The Hard Elements

Sofas, end tables, bookcases, desks, armchairs—these are all the cornerstones of the look and feel of your home. When you purchased these pieces, though, you might have unknowingly brought more into your home than just new furniture. The process of creating furniture can use a lot of toxic chemicals that you do not want in your indoor air.

Pressed Woods

Back in the olden days, furniture was actually made from solid pieces of wood and was built to last for generations. Today, furniture is a lot less costly than it used to be, but that is because of the materials that it can be made from. While solid wood pieces are still available, a majority of affordable furniture is made from pressed woods, which are created by "pressing" bits of wood together and using chemical-laden adhesives to create a seemingly solid sheet of wood. These less expensive materials are often called particleboard, or medium density fiberboard (MDF). The chemicals that are used in the adhesives can off-gas into your indoor air and contribute to poor indoor air quality.

Formaldehyde Exposure

The adhesives that are often used to create pressed woods can contain formaldehyde. Yes, the same stuff that is used to embalm bodies can be used to create your furniture. In fact, the EPA states that in homes, "the most significant sources of formaldehyde are likely to be pressed wood products made using adhesives than contain urea-formaldehyde (UF) resins."

ALERT

Not all pressed woods are made from adhesives that contain formaldehyde, but the majority of them are. There have been a lot of improvements in the market and manufacturers are finding nontoxic solutions to create pressed woods, but look for a label stating that the product is formaldehyde-free or call the manufacturer.

The formaldehyde off-gasses from the furniture, but it isn't a quick process. Off-gassing can last for several years after the product was created. The greatest amounts of formaldehyde, though, are released when the product is new, while increased heat and humidity levels inside your home can make the formaldehyde off-gas even quicker. Unfinished or raw edges of pressed woods, which don't have a sealant or coating on them, will off-gas formaldehyde even more quickly.

Health Risks

Exposure to formaldehyde fumes can lead to many health problems. Some of the health effects may show up immediately, while others may take time to develop. Among the health risks are:

- Burning sensations in the eyes and throat
- Nausea
- Asthma attacks
- Eye, nose, and throat irritation
- Wheezing
- Coughing
- Fatigue
- Skin rash
- Severe allergic reactions
- Cancer

In homes with a significant amount of new products made from pressed woods (which includes furniture, hardwood plywood wall paneling, cabinetry, and built-in shelving), the formaldehyde levels can be greater than three times the level at which humans can start to suffer some health effects.

Fix the Problem

If you have recently bought a new piece of furniture made primarily from pressed woods, see if you can return it. If you recently bought furniture or have new cabinetry made from pressed woods, and removing them from your home is not an option, then increase the air circulation in your home by opening windows and screened doors as frequently as possible to get fresh air in and the formaldehyde out. Keep the temperature and humidity levels inside your home low to prevent the formaldehyde from off-gassing even faster.

When it comes time to buy furniture, solid wood furniture is a great choice, especially unfinished wood. For finished wood pieces, ask if the finishes are nontoxic and formaldehyde-free. Metal furniture, or metal and glass combinations, are a great alternative, too.

ESSENTIAL

If you have had some furniture pieces that are made from pressed woods for several years now, you probably do not need to worry. Chances are the pressed wood has already off-gassed and there is very little formaldehyde still being emitted into the air.

Healthy furniture does not have to cost a lot. Chain stores such as Walmart and Ikea often have affordable nontoxic choices among their selections. Thrift store and antique store finds are also inexpensive. If the pieces are at least several years old, the formaldehyde-containing resins would have off-gassed already. Older furniture also tends to be made with better quality materials, too, such as solid wood.

Furniture—The Soft Elements

The hard structural pieces of a piece of furniture are not the only concern for exposure to toxic chemicals at home. Many of the pieces of furniture that you sit in are also constructed of the soft, cushiony material of polyurethane foam to make your bum more comfortable. Polyurethane foam is actually a petroleum product. Yes, it is made from oil. From a health perspective, polyurethane foam is a major concern because it breaks down easily, disintegrating into tiny particles that become airborne and are inhaled by your family. Polyurethane foam can contain a myriad of chemicals, including formaldehyde (yes, it rears its ugly head again), toluene, benzene, and—of great concern—fire retardants.

ESSENTIAL

Stain-repellent coatings for cushions can contain formaldehyde, with the same health risks as formaldehyde used in pressed woods. Opt out of the coating if buying a product from the manufacturer. If the sales agent does not ask about your preferences, ask if you can buy the product without the coating. Do not apply ready-made stain repellents to anything in your home.

PBDE Fire Retardants

Because polyurethane foam is so flammable, it has to be doused in heavy-duty chemical fire retardants. The most commonly used fire retardants before 2005 were PBDEs, polybrominated diphenyl ethers. These fire retardants don't just stay in the foam, though. They can off-gas and become airborne for years to come. PBDEs are considered a major health concern because so many of us are exposed to them so often, from the padded office chair you sit in every day to the mattress that you sleep on every night. That is why the form of PBDEs that were used in foam furniture was removed from the manufacturing of U.S. household items in 2005. However, many people still use furniture and other items that were bought before the ban, such as couches, chairs, mattresses, pillows, etc.

PBDEs are similar in structure to some banned neurotoxins. The health risks of exposure to PBDEs include:

- Slow brain development
- Hyperactivity
- Behavioral disorders
- Immune suppression
- Endocrine disruption
- Damage of the thyroid and liver
- Cancer

Prevent PBDE Exposure

If you have polyurethane foam cushions that are starting to fall apart and breaking down into small bits and pieces, especially ones made before

2005, it is best to dispose of them. If you cannot get rid of the item, be sure to keep it covered and encased to prevent the small pieces of foam from being inhaled. Vacuuming frequently will keep the small particles from entering your indoor air, as well. Do not buy secondhand furniture that contains polyurethane foam.

When purchasing new furniture with cushions, try to find items made with natural filling materials. Wool is a naturally fire-retardant material, but other natural materials will still need a fire retardant by law. Check with the manufacturer to make sure that these natural fillings have not been treated with unnecessary harsh chemicals. Buy unupholstered products when possible, such as desk chairs or dining room table chairs. You can add cushions on your own. It can be much easier to purchase all-natural cushions or make your own to accommodate your needs, instead of trying to find a manufacturer to do it.

Paints

There is no better way to give a room a total makeover than to apply a new coat of paint. You do not want to add anything more to your room, though, than an updated sense of style. Many paint colors can contain a high amount of volatile organic compounds (VOCs). VOCs are small amounts of potentially toxic chemicals that release from a product into your indoor air. Many paints are full of high levels of VOCs, but there are plenty of options that are not. Preventing an increase of toxic chemicals in your freshly painted room is as easy as picking the right can of color.

Low- and No-VOC Paints

Paint is one of the top VOC exposures for the average homeowner. That new paint smell that you are familiar with? That's off-gassing VOCs. But even after the smell disappears, VOCs can be off-gassing for months, and even years. That is why it is so important to purchase low- or no-VOC paints to reduce your chemical exposure. Low-VOC paints use water as a carrier instead of petroleum-based solvents, and contain very low levels of formaldehyde and heavy metals, such as mercury and cadmium, which are often added to paints but can detach and become part of your indoor air. No-VOC paints contain five grams per liter or less of VOCs.

It is not always as easy as just going to the paint store and picking up a can of low- or no-VOC paint, though. The terms "low-VOC" or "no-VOC" often refer to the VOC content in the base of the paint, not the tint that creates the color. Those tints can really boost the VOC content of paints. Be sure to ask the paint professional if the low- or no-VOC claim is just for the base, or includes the base and tint. If they do not know, go elsewhere. No sense in thinking you are getting a low- or no-VOC product when you're not.

Milk Paints

Milk paints are one of the healthiest color options that you can find for your home. Just like the name implies, milk paints are made from a dried form of natural milk protein. These were the first types of paints ever used, going back as far as caveman times, and have been used ever since. In fact, the colors most often associated with Colonial America furniture and homes were created with milk paints. The simple combination of milk protein, pigment, and lime creates a paint that does not contain any VOCs and has long-lasting color.

FACT

Even the famed King Tutankhamun colored his world of riches with milk paint. When King Tut's tomb was opened in 1924, many items found inside the burial chamber, including models of people and boats, as well as pieces of furniture, had been painted with milk paint.

Reduce Your VOC Exposure

All forms of paint, not just the stuff on your walls, can cause VOC exposures. If you have old cans of paint sitting around in your home, remove them because they can release VOCs even stored in the can. If you are concerned about matching colors, keep the paint can top, or at least the paperwork showing the tint ingredients, so that you can match the color again if needed. If you have recently painted your house, regardless of what type of paint you used, be sure to increase the ventilation and open your windows when possible.

ALERT

Paints need to be disposed of as hazardous waste (that should tell you something!), so do not simply throw them out with your weekly trash. Contact your city or county's government for information on hazardous waste removal or hazardous waste days, or search Earth911.com (*www.earth911.com*) for local disposal centers.

Before choosing a new can of paint, investigate your options first. Low- and no-VOC paints are available at mass retailers, specialty paint stores, and online. If you are concerned about VOCs being added during the tinting process, though, it is wise to pick a paint brand that you want to use, then start choosing colors from there. Some brands offer only specific colors of low-VOC paint. Other brands can color-match a paint sample using their own low-VOC tints, if done at their own store. Always choose latex paint over oil-based paint because it releases fewer toxins. Be sure to properly ventilate any area where you are painting, both during the painting procedure and for weeks afterward.

Window Coverings

There are a myriad of ways to dress up your windows. Not only do curtains, blinds, and shades complete your decorating palette, but they are highly functional in blocking out the light and giving you a little more privacy inside your home. While window treatments can make or break the look of a room, that is really about all of the attention that they get. It is easy to hang some curtains or blinds and forget about them, but that is exactly where the health problems may lie.

Curtains

Think about it. Curtains are just pieces of fabric that are decoratively hung from the wall. You know how dirty and dusty places like dresser tops and shelves can get throughout your home just from air blowing around? Well, curtains are the same way because the fabric traps the dust. To make matters worse, though, curtains are not laundered nearly as often as surfaces might be dusted, so the amount of allergy- and asthma-inducing dust on these accessories can be mind-boggling. The easy, and only, solution is to simply wash your curtains more often. When choosing curtains, make sure that they are made from a material that can be easily laundered. If not, take the curtains outside and beat them with a broom to remove the dust.

Mini Blinds

Mini blinds are an easily affordable window treatment. That is because they are made from inexpensive PVC plastic. When putting plastic materials in windows that are exposed to hot sunlight and harsh UV rays every day, though, you might want to consider the fact that high heat can make plastic break down faster. With the degradation of the plastic materials comes the risk of chemicals being released into your indoor air and into your home.

ESSENTIAL

Since 1990, more than 200 infants and children have been accidentally strangled because of being caught in a mini blind cord. While mini blinds made after 2001 should have safety features, all mini blinds can be retrofitted to become safer. An excellent resource on fixing this child safety hazard, as well as free retrofitting kits, is the Window Covering Safety Council (*www.windowcoverings.org*).

There are some mini blinds that pose a definite health risk, though. Mini blinds manufactured overseas before 1997 were found to have lead added to the plastic. As the mini blinds deteriorate, lead dust is formed and can be inhaled or ingested. If you still have mini blinds from that era, consider removing them from your home and installing new blinds. For overall health and peace of mind, choose blinds made from unfinished bamboo or wood, Roman shades made from cloth, or simple cloth window coverings, instead.

Throw Pillows and Blankets

Just like with curtains, dust and subsequently dust mites can build up in pillows and blankets on the couch or other chairs throughout your home. As a leading cause of allergies and asthma, this accumulation of dust can cause adverse health effects. While bedding in your bedroom might be washed very frequently, it is often easy to overlook the decorative pillows and cozy blankets that might be a staple in your living room or den. Launder pillows and throws frequently, but be careful of washing instructions. Often, decorative elements must be dry-cleaned or hand-washed only. If washing an item in hot water is not feasible, place the item outside in full sun for several hours to naturally kill the dust mites.

Lighting

In the quest for homeowners to become more energy efficient, compact fluorescent light (CFL) bulbs are becoming more widely used. In fact, old-fashioned incandescent bulbs are quickly being phased out while CFL bulbs and light-emitting diodes (LED) lighting are becoming more common. It seems that the only problem associated with CFL bulbs is their use of mercury, and the problems that might arise if a bulb breaks.

FACT

An Energy Star Qualified CFL bulb uses 75 percent less energy than a standard incandescent bulb and can save more than $40 in electricity costs for the lifetime of the bulb. A CFL bulb can last six times longer than an incandescent bulb and produces 75 percent less heat, which also cuts the expense of cooling costs for a home.

Mercury in Lighting

CFLs contain about 1 percent of the amount of mercury found in a mercury thermometer. Even though the amount is small, mercury exposure is a valid health concern because mercury is a neurotoxin. If a CFL lightbulb breaks in your home, a small amount of mercury vapor will be released. The mercury levels around a leak can be quite high for an hour or more unless there is proper ventilation. The mercury that escapes from a CFL can also ball up into tiny beads, which are especially toxic if not handled properly. There are no health risks associated with CFL bulbs unless a bulb breaks.

ALERT

It is important to properly dispose of CFL bulbs in order to prevent mercury exposure to your family and prevent the release of mercury into the environment. CFL bulbs can be recycled, and some states require you to recycle the bulbs. Many national retail chains, such as Ikea and Home Depot, offer CFL recycling stations. The EPA offers links (*www.epa.gov/cfl/cflrecycling.html*) to recycling options.

Preventing Mercury Exposure

Being careful where and when you use a CFL bulb will reduce your risk of accidentally breaking the bulb. Do not put CFL bulbs in lighting fixtures that might easily be knocked over, such as in a child's room or along a busy hallway. Do not install the bulbs in light fixtures with no protection for the bulb. Do not bother installing CFL bulbs in places where the light is not on for more than fifteen minutes, such as in a closet, because CFL bulbs take ten to fifteen minutes to warm up and reach their full lighting potential.

Removing a CFL bulb should always be done carefully. Switch the bulb off and allow it to cool before removing. Handle the bulb by the base, not the glass tubing. Consider putting a drop cloth under a CFL bulb before attempting to remove it in case it should break. If a CFL bulb does break, there are guidelines that you should follow for your family's health. The EWG's "When a Bulb Breaks" (*www.ewg.org/Mercury/CFL-Lightbulbs-When-a-Bulb-Breaks*) highlights the safety measures that should be taken.

Candles

Used in just about every room of the house, candles are not just a source of lighting, but also a way to infuse warmth and atmosphere into your surroundings. Some candles are made from materials that will give off more than just a pleasant fragrance in your home, though. Candles that are made from synthetic ingredients, such as paraffin derived from petroleum, can release chemicals into your indoor air while melting. Candle wicks can be a problem, too, if they contain lead and heavy metals. Candle wicks made from 100 percent cotton are ideal because they do not contain toxic materials.

Artificial Fragrances

Candles are often burned to impart a fragrance, but if the fragrance comes from artificial ingredients, it simply adds to the problems of bad indoor air. An "artificial fragrance" is not just one chemical used to scent a product. As discussed earlier in this book, artificial fragrance is a generic term that is used to identify the presence of up to 3,194 chemicals that have been blended together to make a scent.

Natural Alternatives

Remove any artificially scented candles, including jar candles or gel candles that are stored throughout your home. These include candles on display, as well as candles that might be stored away in a cabinet somewhere. If you are not sure if a candle is artificially scented, assume it is, since the majority of candles available for mass purchase use artificial fragrances. If you have been using artificially fragranced candles, open the windows in your home and really air the place out for at least several hours, if not for a few days.

ESSENTIAL

Beeswax has been used for thousands of years and can be used in lip balms, furniture polishes, soaps, and waterproofing finishes. Beeswax candles burn brighter, longer, and cleaner than any other type of candle. The natural scent of beeswax is created when bees create beeswax honeycombs after pollinating fragrant flowers.

When buying candles, look for ones made from soy wax, beeswax, or palm wax. These all-natural waxes are gentler on your health. Make sure the wick is made of 100 percent cotton, or that the product states that it is lead-free. Look for a product made with only 100 percent essential oil fragrance.

CHECKLIST FOR DECORATING A HEALTHY HOME

❑ Avoid purchasing furniture made from pressed woods, unless made with formaldehyde-free resins. Pressed woods are the major source of exposure to formaldehyde in a person's home. Formaldehyde, a common indoor air pollutant, can cause a variety of health problems ranging from fatigue to cancer.

❑ Dispose of foam cushions and furniture that are starting to break apart and deteriorate. Foam cushions can release toxic chemical fire retardants into your indoor air, which are then inhaled.

❑ Choose low- or no-VOC options of paint. Reduce your exposure to many indoor air contaminants by choosing paints that do not contain as many of the health offenders.

❑ Do not use CFL bulbs in light fixtures that could easily be knocked over. Because mercury is found in a CFL bulb, you want to ensure that the bulb will not accidentally break.

❑ Do not use stain repellents, and decline the option when purchasing furniture. Stain repellents contain the same types of chemicals as some fire retardants and can build up in your body's tissues.

❑ Air out your home for several weeks after painting with any type of paint. Even low- and no-VOC paints can still contain small amounts of pollutants, so bringing fresh air indoors can reduce your indoor air pollution.

❑ If a CFL bulb breaks, follow the proper procedures to clean the mercury spill. Leave the room after breakage to reduce your exposure to inhaling mercury, a neurotoxin, and contain the toxic material with special care.

❑ Wash your curtains regularly. Dust, dust mites, and allergens can build up in the fabric.

❑ Dispose of any mini blinds manufactured before 1997. Older mini blinds have been found to contain lead in the plastic.

❑ Only burn candles made from natural waxes and essential oils with a lead-free wick. Candles made of synthetic ingredients release chemicals into your indoor air, while lead-based wicks allow the toxic metal to be inhaled.

CHAPTER 7

Flooring

You walk on it, your kids play on it, and your dog even sleeps on it. Your family has a lot more interaction with your home's flooring than you might think. In the grand scheme of things in your house, your flooring might not get much attention, but it can have a major impact on your health. In fact, choosing the right type of flooring and keeping it properly cleaned can dramatically reduce some common respiratory ailments while also contributing to a much healthier home.

What Flooring Will Work Best for You?

When your floors start to get worn and dirty, you might just try to look the other way or buy a throw rug for the problem since replacing flooring is such a major task. Perhaps you are in the process of building or refurbishing a home and you must purchase new flooring. Maybe you are just tired of your old flooring or wondering if some of your health problems could be caused from the flooring that you currently have. Whatever situation you might be in, it is helpful to know what the appropriate type of flooring is for your family's specific needs in order to minimize health problems down the road.

Types of Flooring

Several decades ago, the choices in home flooring were pretty dismal. Times have clearly changed. Today's technological achievements now allow anyone to choose from among a wide range of flooring materials in all kinds of price ranges, which include:

- **Wall-to-wall carpeting.** Adding a little cushion underneath every step that you take, wall-to-wall carpeting is a solid sheet of carpeting that extends to every wall within a room. A pad is necessary underneath the carpeting.
- **Hardwood floors.** Made of planks of one solid piece of wood, hardwood floors can be expensive. You can purchase prefinished hardwood floors, or unfinished wood floors and apply a protective finish on-site.
- **Engineered hardwood floors.** If you like the look of wood floors, but not the price, engineered hardwood floors offer a more economical solution by laminating several pieces of hardwood together.
- **Laminate.** Designed to look like wood or stone without the hefty expense, laminate flooring is often a very affordable flooring choice. Made up of many layers, laminate is often composed of synthetic resins and fiberboard.
- **Stone.** Natural slabs of stone such as granite, marble, and slate create a long-lasting floor that might be much more costly than some other options.

- **Tile.** Often made of ceramic or glass, tile flooring is installed with grout and creates a hard surface.
- **Vinyl.** Among the most economical flooring choices, peel-and-stick vinyl tiles are extremely easy to install and come in a wide array of colors and styles.
- **Linoleum.** Made with just linseed oil, cork dust, wood flour, resins, and pigments, linoleum is making a comeback because of its non-toxic, green ingredients.
- **Cork.** Just like the corkboards you push thumbtacks into, cork flooring comes from the bark of cork oak trees and can dampen sounds just like carpeting.
- **Bamboo.** Similar to hardwood floors, bamboo flooring is made of strips of rapidly renewable bamboo grass.

There are often different types of flooring within each category, too. For instance, if you choose hardwood floors, you will then need to decide whether you would like domestic wood or exotic hardwoods. Within each category there might also be healthier options of some materials compared to others. For example, bamboo flooring made with formaldehyde resins would have more health concerns than bamboo flooring made with non-toxic resins.

Flooring for Lifestyle Needs

Only you can decide what type of flooring is appropriate for your family and your home. No two homeowners are alike, so you shouldn't choose flooring just because it looks good in someone else's house. There is no sense in adding more drama and cleaning into your everyday life if you do not have to. For example, do you have large dogs that run in the field each day before coming inside the house? Then white carpeting is definitely not ideal for you, unless you enjoy plenty of hard labor on a daily basis. Are there moisture control issues in your basement? Then do not try to use wooden floors, which will end up warped and ruined. Trying to minimize the noise level in a certain room? You will only drive yourself crazy if you choose a stone floor instead of carpeting.

Flooring for Health and Safety

You should always consider your family's health and behavioral patterns before narrowing down your flooring choices. If you have young kids or are planning a family in the future, laying stone or ceramic tile in the living room will not be too kind when your kids are learning to walk and falling down quite often. Have older parents with mobility issues? Carpeting might be better to prevent falling, but if your parents use a wheelchair, you will want to use flooring that allows better maneuverability. If any member of your family has issues with allergies or asthma, you will want to choose a hypoallergenic flooring option that will not release chemicals or harbor dirt or debris.

Pros and Cons of Flooring Materials

While style, color, and ease of cleaning are major factors in choosing flooring, so are potential health hazards associated with a flooring material, as well as environmental concerns in your home that would create unfavorable conditions for certain materials. The following table highlights the pros and cons of specific types of flooring:

▼ PROS AND CONS OF FLOORING MATERIALS

Type of Floor	Pros	Cons
Carpet	Soft, slip-resistant	Absorbs spills, prone to staining, not great for allergies, can allow mold to grow, VOC exposure
Hardwood	Durable, easily refinished	Liquids can damage, humidity levels can make floor strips move, must be installed above ground level
Bamboo	Can be refinished, some are very durable	Some can be easily scratched and dented, can crack or warp with significant humidity change
Laminate and vinyl	Spills are easily wiped away, will not scratch or dent easily	VOC exposure can aggravate asthma and allergies
Stone and tile	Spills are easily wiped away, antimicrobial	Hard surface can be painful for falls, acids can cause damage
Linoleum	Antimicrobial, antistatic, hypoallergenic, spills are easily wiped away	Cannot be refinished
Cork	Soft, sound-absorbent, hypoallergenic, antimicrobial, antistatic	May move with humidity changes

Choosing a flooring material is not something that should be done quickly just because a store is having a three-day sale. Flooring can be a major expense, so you do not want to have to install a new floor several years down the road after you find out that your first choice wasn't a great fit for your home or your family. With so many potential health hazards associated with certain flooring materials, as well, a little bit of research and thought can go a long way in creating a healthier home.

Anatomy of a Carpet

If you walk into a room that has just had carpet installed, chances are you notice a "new carpet smell." That telltale smell is actually an indicator of just how many toxic fumes are being released into the air from all of the chemicals used in the manufacturing of carpet. A typical sample of carpet can contain as many as 120 chemicals. When choosing a healthier carpet for your home, you have to investigate every single component of the carpeting before making your choice to ensure that you are indeed receiving the non-toxic carpet that you are striving for.

ESSENTIAL

Both the EPA and the CPSC suggest that before you have new carpet installed, you should have the retailer unroll and air out the carpet in a well-ventilated area before installation, ask for low-emitting adhesives, and leave the house during the installation, as well as for several hours afterward.

Fibers

Carpeting is made using a process called tufting. Tufting is the act of looping many, many fibers through a backing material to create a carpet. Those fibers can be made of different types of materials, but in the U.S. carpet industry, more than 99 percent of those materials are synthetic. The majority of U.S. carpets are made of one of these four fibers:

- Nylon
- Olefin (polypropylene)

- Acrylic
- Polyester

Since almost all wall-to-wall carpeting manufactured in the United States is made of synthetic materials, VOCs being released from the fibers is a very real concern. Because the materials are made primarily from chemicals, small amounts of those chemicals can be released into your home's indoor air from the carpeting over the course of many months or several years.

Natural carpet fibers, such as wool, cotton, jute, and coir, will not release VOCs unless they have been treated with a synthetic chemical finish. Wool is also naturally fire-resistant, dust-mite resistant, antimicrobial, and repels stains and liquids. An excellent source for 100 percent wool carpeting made in the United States is Earth Weave Carpet Mills (*www.earthweave.com*).

Since wool is such a great all-around choice for a healthier carpet, why isn't it used more often? Quite honestly, it is because of the cost. Wool must come from sheep who are raised for the fiber, taking time and expense to take care for the herds, while synthetic chemicals can quickly and easily be created in a factory anywhere.

ESSENTIAL

To find carpeting made of any kind of fiber that is low in VOC emissions, look for the Carpet and Rug Institute's (*www.carpet-rug.org*) Green Label or Green Label Plus. The program identifies carpets, cushions, and adhesives that have met stringent indoor air-quality requirements for very low VOC emissions.

Padding

Even if you purchased a carpet made from all-natural fibers, you could still be exposing yourself to high amounts of VOCs through the padding that is put underneath the carpet to make it soft. Formaldehyde is a chemical used often in carpet padding. Styrene-butadiene rubber (SBR) is often used in carpet padding, too, and can off-gas many VOCs. Natural and nontoxic padding, such as felt, jute, or natural rubber, is available for carpets, but not widely used, so you would need to ask for it specifically.

Chemical Finishes

Synthetic fibers need to be doused with chemical fire retardants because they are highly flammable. Carpet fibers of any kind, though, whether synthetic or natural, may be coated with a number of other chemical-based finishes for a variety of reasons. Many carpets are manufactured with a stain repellent to help prevent spills from absorbing into the carpet fibers. Carpet could also be coated with fungicides, antimicrobial agents, mothproofing, and antistatic treatments. Even if your carpet is made of all-natural materials, but doused in chemical finishes, it is not as healthy as you might think. In fact, a synthetic carpet without any finishes might be more healthy than a wool carpet coated with everything that could possibly be added to the carpet fiber. The more finishes that are on your carpet, the more VOCs that will off-gas into your home's indoor air.

Hard Flooring

There are plenty more flooring options other than carpeting. In fact, if you do not choose carpeting, you might be confused and overwhelmed with all of the options that are now available. All of these floors are relatively easy to clean with simple sweeping and mopping, but the similarities end there.

Hardwood Flooring

Hardwood flooring, whether solid wood, engineered wood, or bamboo, is a flooring option that can stand the test of time. Centuries-old houses often still retain their original solid wood floors that, with a little refinishing, are still as good as new.

When using solid wood or bamboo, you do not have to be as concerned with what synthetic materials were used in the production of the flooring because the flooring comes straight from nature. While the materials might be all natural, you do still have to be concerned about finishes that are applied to the wood or bamboo. If you install unfinished wood or bamboo flooring, you can apply finishes yourself, which allows you to be in control about what is added to your floors.

Engineered wood is a little different. Since engineered wood consists of many layers of wood held together by an adhesive, you must be careful about what chemicals are in the adhesive if you want to reduce your chemical exposure. Formaldehyde is one example of a chemical that is often added to adhesives that are used with engineered woods.

Laminate wood flooring is also available, though it cannot really be compared to floors made primarily of wood and bamboo. Laminate flooring is synthetic and has a resin-infused paper topcoat that is actually a picture of wood and looks amazingly the same. Underneath is a thick layer of wood composite. With all of the resins and adhesives used in this flooring material, the chances of chemicals being off-gassed are very high, and you must still be concerned with formaldehyde exposure.

ALERT

The only way to know for sure if flooring contains formaldehyde that can off-gas into your home's indoor air is to look for products labeled "formaldehyde-free." If you do not see a label, call or e-mail the manufacturer directly to learn more about what is used in the resins and finishes of the product.

Linoleum and Vinyl Floors

Linoleum is often confused with vinyl flooring. The two can look the same, though they each have very different health impacts. Vinyl flooring is synthetic and made with PVC and chlorinated petrochemicals. Vinyl can off-gas many different VOCs into your indoor air. Linoleum, on the other hand, is the exact opposite. Made with simple, all-natural materials such as linseed oil, limestone, wood flour, cork dust, tree resins, and pigments, linoleum will not release VOCs into your home's indoor air.

FACT

Linoleum was patented in 1863 by Frederick Walton. He got the idea from the skin of oxidized linseed oil that forms on paint. Named after the Latin words of *linum* (the word for flax, where linseed oil comes from) and *oleum* (the word for oil), the original recipe that Walton created is still used by linoleum makers today.

Linoleum used to be considered an old-fashioned flooring option that you would never consider adding to your home. Highly popular in the early and mid-twentieth century, linoleum once lost its luster but is now making a serious comeback as a nontoxic flooring option with style appeal. Linoleum costs about the same as vinyl flooring, making it a highly affordable healthy flooring option. It has natural antimicrobial properties that inhibit the growth of dust mites and bacteria, as well as natural antistatic properties that repel dust and dirt.

Vinyl flooring is readily available in mass retailers and flooring supply centers. Linoleum is easily found, too. Forbo Flooring Systems (*www .forbo-flooring.us/Residential-Flooring/Products*) is the world's leader in linoleum floor coverings and sells more than half of the world's linoleum. Their Marmoleum flooring comes in an entire rainbow of colors, with more than 120 options of Marmoleum sheet flooring. Armstrong (*www.armstrong.com*) offers linoleum flooring options, too.

Cork

Want a softer surface for your floors, but concerned about the health effects of carpeting? Cork is a great option for you. Cork flooring is made of the bark of the cork oak tree, the same type of material that creates wine bottle stoppers and corkboards. The bark can be harvested from the tree without cutting it down, creating a long-lasting resource for flooring materials.

FACT

Famed architect Frank Lloyd Wright chose cork flooring for use in many of his designs, including the legendary Fallingwater residence in Pennsylvania. The U.S. Department of Commerce building, the Department of the Interior building, the National Archives, and the Mayo Clinic all had cork flooring in the early 1900s, when cork flooring was highly popular and widely used.

Cork flooring has many positive benefits compared to other hard flooring options. Cork is composed of 80 percent air, so if something is dropped or moved across a cork tile, the cork will give instead of being scratched or gouged like other materials. Cork is not easily stained, and just requires mopping with soap and water to be cleaned. With its great sound-dampening qualities, cork is ideal for rooms in which you would like to reduce the noise of walking across the floors. The natural flooring material is long-lasting, as well, and can be a beautiful fixture in your home for up to eighty years if properly maintained. Cork does need to be finished with a wax or coating, so ask the manufacturer whether the finish is nontoxic.

Cork flooring is not a one-shade-fits-all kind of cork, unlike corkboards. Cork comes in a wide variety of earth tone shades and style variations, with colors achieved by baking the material, not by using dyes or stains. Cork can be purchased at mass retailers, such as Home Depot (*www.homedepot .com*), Lowe's (*www.lowes.com*), and Lumber Liquidators (*www.lumber liquidators.com*), as well as through manufacturers such as Expanko (*www .expanko.com*).

Stone and Tiles

Stone and tiles create a very hard flooring surface that can be dramatic to look at. These materials can be hard on the feet, joints, and other body parts, though, especially if you walk barefoot throughout the house or have small children who run and fall. Installed with grout to keep the stone and tile attached to the floor, you must be careful when cleaning the flooring because certain cleaners can lead to discoloration of the grout. Cleaning agents such as soap and vinegar, the staples of nontoxic cleaning, can actually damage stone and grout, which makes it harder to clean your floors on your own terms. Instead, you will be tied down to a specialty cleaner manufactured solely for stone and tile floors.

Laminate stone and tile flooring is an option, too, if you want the look of stone or tile without the expense. Just like with laminate wood flooring, though, you must be careful about the resins and adhesives used in the creation of the materials. Laminate is typically not a low-VOC option, and formaldehyde exposure is possible.

Area Rugs

Though area rugs can harbor the same health hazards that room-by-room carpeting does, there is one big difference: Area rugs can easily be taken outside and laundered. The ability to remove the carpet and clean it and allow it to dry outside of your home is a big plus when comparing the health hazards of carpeting. Area rugs offer you the cushiness and sound-dampening qualities of carpeting with the ease and convenience of being able to clean them and replace them however and whenever you would like.

Area rugs are more likely to be made from natural materials, such as sisal, seagrass, jute, coir, wool, and cotton, although the majority are still made from synthetic materials. Area rugs do not necessarily need padding, either, which further reduces your exposure to synthetic carpeting materials.

Cleaning

Whether you have a small carpeted runner for the hallway or a massive area rug under the dining room table, make sure that it can easily be removed. For instance, do not nail the rug down into the flooring underneath or glue it into place. If the rug is not portable, it defeats the whole purpose of buying an area rug.

When choosing an area rug, pay attention to laundering directions for the rug. Does the rug need to be dry-cleaned? If so, how often do you think that you will actually take it to the dry cleaners and how much is it going to cost each time that you do? Large area rugs are not going to be able to fit into a standard washing machine at home, so even if they are able to be washed, how and where will you take them? Smaller rugs for the kitchen and bath should easily be able to run through your wash at home. If dry-cleaning or the washing machine is not an option, you can always bring the rugs outside and hose them off or beat them to remove dirt and debris. Allowing the rug to stay in full sun for several hours will naturally kill dust mites and disinfect the rug at no cost to you.

ESSENTIAL

There are actually tools called carpet beaters or rug beaters that are designed to properly beat a rug to release the dirt and debris that builds up over time. If you do not want to purchase a rug beater, you could also use a broom handle, tennis racket, badminton racket, or large stick to clean the rug outside.

Safety

Regardless of what size or type of area rug that you choose, it is essential that the rug has a nonslip coating underneath to prevent accidental falls and injuries. Many rugs come with a nonstick coating in place on the underside of the rug. However, smaller rugs made of cloth, sisal, or other woven materials often do not. Purchase a nonslip pad to put underneath every single rug in your home that does not have a nonslip backing and make sure that the rug does not move around under foot. Adhesive nonslip strips can also be purchased to apply directly to the underside of the rug.

Existing Flooring

After reading about all of the potential pitfalls of flooring options, you might be worried about the floors that you have had in your home for many years. While new flooring and refinishing floors will release the most chemicals and VOCs into your home, there are some things to consider when talking about old flooring, too.

If you have had your carpet for at least three years, most of the off-gassing will have already occurred. The highest amounts of VOCs will off-gas within the first three months of bringing a new carpet into your home. Lower amounts of VOCs can still be released into your home's air for two or three more years. After that time frame, your main concern should be on cleaning and mold control, instead of VOC exposure. Vinyl floors and other flooring materials have similar off-gassing time frames. If you have had your flooring for several years, then VOC exposure will be minimal compared to VOCs coming off of freshly installed flooring.

When the time comes to remove flooring for any reason, you must be extremely careful. Old flooring could have been manufactured with materials that are now known safety hazards. Old vinyl floor tiles could contain asbestos, which was commonly used to strengthen the flooring many years ago. Old painted wooden floors might contain lead from lead-based paint that was used several decades ago. Carpet padding made before 2005 could have been manufactured with polyurethane foam that was treated with PBDEs, a toxic chemical fire retardant. Not only do you need to worry about the materials that were once allowed to be used in the manufacturing of the flooring, but you also need to be aware of what might have built up underneath the flooring ever since, such as mold and layers of dust.

ALERT

For health and safety reasons for your entire family, it is often best to hire a professional who is certified to properly remove the type of flooring that you have and deal with any health hazards if they arise, such as lead or asbestos removal.

There is no one way to properly remove all flooring. Carpeting could be attached to either hardwood floors or concrete. Tiles might be attached to mortar underneath. Removing flooring is a difficult task that is only made more difficult by not knowing for sure what is located underneath. You must consider the flooring that you are removing, what it is attached to, what toxic materials it might contain, and the best way to prevent any chemical exposure into the rest of your home. You can remove flooring by yourself if you properly investigate the techniques for your specific situation, seal off the area to prevent any health hazards from migrating into the rest of your home, and are ready for some heavy manual labor.

CHECKLIST FOR HEALTHY FLOORS

❑ Consider your family's health needs when purchasing new flooring. Certain floors are beneficial for people with allergies or other special needs. Because flooring is in every room of the house, it is vital to consider how it will affect a person's health and choose options that fit your needs.

❑ If you have had new flooring installed in the past two years, especially vinyl or laminate options, make sure you have proper ventilation throughout your home. You can reduce your exposure to off-gassing chemicals coming from new flooring materials or adhesives by increasing ventilation throughout your home.

❑ Clean rugs routinely. To reduce the amount of dust, allergens, and chemical buildup that occurs in carpet fibers, it is important to clean them regularly.

❑ Ensure that rugs have nonslip surfaces underneath. Rugs that easily move underfoot are a safety risk.

❑ Do not stress over flooring that has been in your home for more than two to three years unless you are experiencing health problems. Chances are, older flooring has released a majority of the pollutants that it contained when installed.

CHAPTER 8

Kitchen

The kitchen is usually the one room in the house where healthy habits start, but there can be a hidden, dangerous side to your kitchen, too. Some of the common products that you use to prepare meals can actually be undoing all of the positive health benefits that you are striving for by eating right. The good news? It is easy to make a few changes that will lead to an even healthier life. Even better, there's no cutting calories or giving up savory foods in this easy kitchen makeover.

Nonstick Cookware

Unless you are just cooking microwave meals every night, you must have some pots and pans around the house. You might have quite an assortment of nonstick cookware, from baking sheets and muffin tins to frying pans and stockpots, since nonstick cookware is so common. With the promises of less time spent on cleanup and fewer calories consumed without the need of oils and shortening, trying to find cookware without nonstick coatings can be a little challenging. Yet for all of the promises of making our life better and easier, nonstick cookware might have a dark side.

PFCs

Pots and pans are called "nonstick" when they have been coated with a material known as polytetrafluorotheylene (PTFE). This synthetic substance is also known as Teflon. PTFE is considered a perfluorochemical, or PFC. Do not be overwhelmed by this alphabet soup of chemical names, though. The problem is that when nonstick pans are heated at high temperatures, toxic fumes can be released. It does not take long to get to the high heat temperature when these toxic fumes can be released from the nonstick coating. In fact, it can take just two to five minutes on a conventional stovetop before toxic fumes start entering the air.

FACT

PFCs are not only in nonstick cookware. The chemicals are used in stain repellents, too. To avoid exposure, do not use a stain-repellent treatment on carpets or furniture. When ordering new furniture or flooring, ask that the manufacturer does not apply an optional stain repellent. Also, do not purchase clothing with stain or water repellents.

Dangerous Fumes

The fumes released from nonstick pans can have some serious side effects, from killing pet birds to causing flu-like symptoms in humans. Unfortunately, PFCs have been linked with:

- Smaller birth weight
- Elevated cholesterol levels
- Abnormal thyroid hormone levels
- A weaker immune system
- Early menopause

PFCs have been found present in the bodies of almost all Americans, since the chemicals have become so prevalent throughout society. Reducing your exposure when you can will limit the amount of PFCs accumulating in your body.

Increased Exposure

Anyone can be exposed to PFCs in fumes from nonstick cookware. But there are times when you might be even more at risk. Look at your nonstick pots and pans. Do they have small scratches and scrapes in the nonstick coating already? Scratched nonstick coatings are quite common. The problem is that when the coating is damaged in any way, such as with a small nick or scratch, the structural integrity of the coating is compromised. When the coating is not operating as it should, you might be at even more risk of exposure to PFCs.

How to Ditch the Nonstick

To avoid exposure to PFCs and other chemicals found in nonstick coatings, it is easiest to simply avoid nonstick cookware. Go through your kitchen and dispose of as much nonstick cookware that you can while still being able to cook your meals in the meantime. Consider any nonstick baking pans, cake pans, muffin tins, fry pans, woks, pots, and even cooking utensils with a nonstick coating. If you must use nonstick cookware, use the lowest heat possible to cook the food. Also, be sure to run the exhaust fan on your stove if it vents to the outside. Avoid using utensils that might scratch or damage the nonstick coating.

When choosing new cookware, what kind of pots and pans are the safest and healthiest to buy? Stainless steel, glass, and cast iron. Stainless steel and cast iron cookware items are typically easy to find in any cooking aisle and can be much less expensive than the ones with a nonstick coating.

Ceramic cookware is also an option, as long as the glaze does not contain lead. Also be sure to choose stainless steel cooking utensils that do not have a nonstick coating.

ALERT

You might find cookware touting its benefits of being "green nonstick" or "not nonstick." Keep in mind that these new substances have not been around for a long time and therefore long-term studies on their safety have not been done, either. Do your research and decide the safest alternatives for your individual needs.

What should you do about food sticking to your pots and pans? There is nothing wrong with using oil when cooking to prevent food from sticking to the pans. Do not fear using a little olive oil when sautéing some vegetables. It is a heart-healthy fat that can be good for you in moderation, depending on your medical condition. Same goes for coconut oil or other healthier fats that supply necessary nutrients into your diet. Still not convinced or absolutely cannot add oils to your diet? Then try cast iron cookware. It requires no oils or sprays at all, and food will not stick to the pans.

Plastics in the Kitchen

If you open up your kitchen cabinets and cupboards, you will probably find a lot of plastic storage containers, cutlery, serving pieces, plates, cups, and cutting boards lurking inside. Kitchen items made of plastic are often less expensive, less prone to breakage, and come in all kinds of shapes and colors. Yet for all of the convenience that plastic offers us, there is a lot that we do not yet know about how plastics in the kitchen can directly affect our health. It is surprising to realize that just a generation or two ago, plastic items were not that common in homes. Our grandparents did not have plastic water bottles to carry around their drinks all day. Our parents certainly did not have plastic storage containers with coordinating lids that could collapse to create more space in the cupboards. As a child, you probably did not have as much contact with plastic food service items as your children do today.

How could some plastics pose health threats to your family? Certain chemicals used to make some plastic products can leach out of the product into the food or drink stored inside. When you consume the food or drink that has been stored in those plastic containers, you unknowingly consume those chemicals.

Not Enough Studies

As rapidly as the plastics industry has expanded to create new and improved items for the kitchen, the testing and safety data has not been able to keep up. How do you test for the safety of a product over the course of a lifespan when products have not even been around that long? Unfortunately, there has not been enough substantial, long-term research to understand what chemicals you are exposing yourself to by eating, drinking, and cooking with plastic items. Plastic kitchen products are composed of many different chemicals, and we are constantly exposing them to high heat (whether in the dishwasher, with hot foods, or in the microwave), freezing temperatures, and lots of wear and tear.

ESSENTIAL

A plastic item labeled "microwave safe" simply means that the product will not warp, melt, or break at high temperatures in the microwave. It does not mean that the product has been tested for toxins leaching into your foods at the high cooking temperatures of a microwave.

Plastic Alternatives

More than half of all plastics are considered safe for use with food and drink. Plastics number one, two, four, and five do not contain the toxic chemicals that are causing concern in other types of plastics. If you would like to continue to use plastics in the kitchen, these are the numbers that you want to see on your plastic items.

If you do not feel comfortable using plastics of any kind, there are plenty of alternatives for food and drink storage. Stainless steel and glass are time-tested materials that do not leach chemicals into your food or drink and are relatively easy to find in stores. Ceramic containers without a glaze containing lead are also a nontoxic choice.

Making the Switch

Trying to replace all of the plastic products in your kitchen can be a daunting task, not to mention an expensive one. Choosing to replace the most important pieces of your kitchen first and moving on to others later can help you stay within a budget. First, dispose of plastics of any kind that have chips or scratches. Chips and scratches damage the structural integrity of the plastic. Second, replace plastic items that come in contact with hot foods and beverages, such as soup ladles, strainers, soup bowls, and food storage containers.

Next, focus on items that you use every day, whether or not they come into contact with hot food, such as plates, bowls, cutlery, cups, pitchers, and other food storage containers. Finally, do not stress too much about the items that you have in the kitchen that are rarely used, such as a chip and dip bowl you only bring out once a year for a football party or a serving platter that only gets used to display cookies at Christmas. If these items are damaged or showing wear and tear, that is a good sign to replace them. If you rarely use an item, especially if it is not subjected to high heat, you are going to have very little exposure to any possible chemicals during the course of its use.

Avoiding BPA

Bisphenol-A (BPA) is one of the most talked about chemicals in plastic. You probably had not even heard of BPA ten years ago, but now it is a substance that you might be passionate about avoiding. There have been many studies in recent years about this synthetic estrogen that is used in the production of polycarbonate plastics, which are the hard, shatterproof plastic water bottles that are made to stand up to tough conditions. BPA can also be found in epoxy resins, which are the smooth, plastic-like coating inside of a can. Epoxy resins are often found in canned foods and stainless-steel water bottles that have an interior plastic coating.

FACT

More than six billion pounds of BPA are produced annually. BPA is rapidly accumulating in our public waterways, as the chemical is released into the environment through the production of BPA, as well as the disposal of products containing BPA, because BPA-containing plastics cannot be easily recycled and accumulate in landfills.

Proven Health Risks

What is the big deal about BPA? Exposure to the chemical has been linked to some serious health problems such as:

- Obesity
- Diabetes
- Heart disease
- Reduced fertility
- Early puberty
- Thyroid problems
- Increases in certain types of cancer, such as ovarian and prostate cancers

More than 93 percent of Americans have detectable levels of BPA in their urine. When BPA enters the body, it starts to mimic, block, or otherwise interfere with your hormones, such as testosterone, estrogen, and thyroid hormones. When BPA starts acting like a hormone, the normal balance of your body might be thrown off. There are a wide variety of hormones that help your body with reproduction, energy levels, growth and development, and other body systems that BPA might possibly affect.

How BPA Gets into You

How are you exposed to BPA? The chemical can leach into the food or drink from plastic containers that were made with BPA or metal cans that are coated with a resin that contains BPA. Your water, canned green beans, and even your chicken soup could be serving up an unknown dose of a potentially toxic chemical. Studies have shown that BPA will start to leach into water that has been contained in a polycarbonate bottle for twenty-four hours. When these BPA-containing polycarbonate bottles were exposed to high heat, though, the rate of exposure was fifty-five times higher.

ALERT

BPA is not only found in kitchen items. In a study of retail store receipts made from thermal paper, the BPA levels on the receipt were 250 to 1,000 times greater than the amount of BPA typically found in a can of food. BPA can transfer from the paper to your skin and be absorbed into your body.

Banning BPA at Home

While you might be scared about the potentially toxic health effects of BPA, it is surprisingly easy to reduce your exposure to BPA if you know what to look for. BPA is only found in plastics with a recycling number seven. But not all number seven plastics contain BPA, because the number seven category of plastics is a catch-all category that contains many different types of plastic that do not fit anywhere else. Unless you know for sure that the number seven plastics that you use for food or water use are BPA-free, you should remove them from your kitchen. This includes water bottles, cups, food storage containers, utensils, bowls, plates, sippy cups, and baby bottles.

When purchasing a water bottle, choose stainless steel with no plastic or resin coating on the inside. Stainless steel has been proven to be the safest material over time and can be just as easy to clean and carry. Glass bottles are a healthy option, too, and come in many varieties that have protective barriers to prevent them from breaking. If you are concerned about odors or being able to properly clean a stainless steel water bottle, choose a model that can be put into the dishwasher and has a larger mouth for easier cleaning. If you would rather use a plastic water bottle, purchase one that states it is BPA-free or is made with a safer plastic such as number one, two, or five.

Reduce your use of canned foods. Epoxy resins lining the inside of cans of fruit, vegetables, soups, etc., can contain BPA. Choose fresh or frozen foods. If you must eat canned foods, choose manufacturers that do not use an epoxy resin to coat the inside of the can, but there are very few companies that can actually claim a BPA-free can.

Avoiding Polyvinyl Chloride (PVC)

Polyvinyl chloride (PVC) is a plastic that you might have heard of for use in plumbing pipes. You might not have realized that it can be used in kitchen items as well. PVC plastic has many uses, from pipes and siding for buildings to wall and floor coverings. When PVC is used in applications in the kitchen, chemicals must be added to make the plastic soft and flexible instead of hard and rigid like in plumbing pipes.

How PVC Harms

The chemicals added to PVC to make it soft and flexible are the ones that can cause health problems. Known as plasticizers, these chemicals can be made with phthalates. Some phthalates are suspected carcinogens and, just like BPA, are considered hormone disruptors, causing:

- Hormonal abnormalities
- Thyroid disorders
- Birth defects
- Reproductive problems

Producing PVC, as well as incinerating or burning it, releases toxic chemicals called dioxins. You don't want to be exposed to dioxins, since dioxin is the most potent carcinogen known. Since PVC is nearly impossible to recycle, the chemical just keeps adding up in the landfills and leaching into the environment.

PVC Exposure

Just like BPA, the phthalates can easily leach out of the plastic into food or drink stored in a container made with PVC. Especially problematic is the fact that heat, as well as the fat found in foods, are believed to cause these chemicals to leach out at a faster rate. Ironically, plastic wraps, some of which are made with PVC, are designed to be in direct contact with food under these same conditions. Packaged meats, which almost always contain fat, are often wrapped with PVC-containing plastic wrap. Plastic wrap is often placed directly on food in the microwave, which is exposed to high heat, in order to prevent splatters.

FACT

More than 14 billion pounds of PVC are manufactured every year. More than 7 seven billion pounds of PVC plastics are thrown out each year in the United States. Only about one quarter of 1 percent of that amount, which is approximately 18 million pounds, is ever recycled.

Cutting Out PVC

PVC is only found in plastics with a number three recycling symbol. Go through your kitchen cabinets and find any plastic food storage containers that have a number three recycling symbol on them. Other items that might contain PVC in your kitchen include plastic wrap, zip-top plastic bags, and oven bags. You will have to read the packages of these items or call the manufacturer to find out if plastic containing PVC is used. It is a common question and if the manufacturer cannot tell you if PVC is used, find one who can.

When purchasing meat from grocery stores or butcher shops, look for stores that offer fresh-cut meat that has not been pre-packaged in plastic wrap. These departments use butcher paper instead to wrap up your meat as you select it. If your only option is to purchase meat that is wrapped in plastic wrap, keep in mind that not all plastic wraps necessarily contain PVC. Even so, remove the plastic wrap from the meat as soon as you get home. Store the meat in PVC-free plastic bags or glass or stainless steel containers. Wondering what to use to cover food when microwaving? Opt for a paper towel or a reusable food splatter cover specifically made for microwave use.

Avoiding Polystyrene

Polystyrene is another plastic that you might not want around your kitchen. Polystyrene is in the number six plastics category. It can be a thick, solid white foam, often referred to as Styrofoam, or it can look like any other standard plastic. Polystyrene is most often used in disposable plastic items, such as coffee cups, takeout containers, disposable plates, egg cartons, meat trays, and portable coolers.

Polystyrene can take up to 900 years for the plastic to break down in the environment. The plastic is difficult to recycle, too, with few facilities offering polystyrene recycling, even though it is a recyclable, so it just keeps accumulating in our landfills and the environment.

A Cancer-Causing Substance

Polystyrene is made with styrene, a suspected carcinogen, which means it could cause cancer. Just like BPA and PVC, styrene can leach out of a plastic at high temperatures. That fact is especially problematic since polystyrene is most often used in disposable cups to contain hot liquids and plastic to-go boxes in which hot meals are often placed for restaurant takeout.

Eliminating Polystyrene

Go through your kitchen cabinets and dispose of any food or drink storage containers that have a number six recycling symbol on them, including insulated cups, takeout containers you might be reusing, as well as disposable plates, utensils, and cups.

Starbucks is encouraging patrons to use reusable cups, and the company's goal is to have 25 percent of their beverages served in reusable cups by the year 2015. They have a long way to go, though. In 2010, less than 2 percent of beverages were served in reusable cups, accounting for more than 36 million beverages.

Avoid using insulated disposable cups for hot liquids (or any liquids, for that matter). Use a reusable mug, glass, or water bottle at the office, a coffeehouse, or on-the-go. Do not use disposable plates, cups, or cutlery made with polystyrene. If you must use disposable items, look into using products made from healthier and more eco-friendly alternatives, such as bamboo or cornstarch, that are becoming more widely available at mass retailers.

If possible, avoid getting takeout in disposable containers made with plastic number six. Many restaurants have already made the switch to more earth-friendly containers. If you cannot avoid hot takeout foods in polystyrene containers, remove the food as soon as possible once you get to your location and never reheat food in the container.

Buy meat from butcher shops or grocery stores that use butcher paper instead of polystyrene meat trays. If you cannot purchase meat from a store that wraps their meats in butcher paper, remove the meat from the plastic tray as soon as you get home. Never heat or defrost meat in a polystyrene tray.

Proper Food Storage

It does not really matter how safe the container is that you drink out of or store food in if the food is not stored properly. Unless stored at the proper temperature, perishable food can become too warm and cause food to spoil, resulting in health problems from food-borne illnesses. Foods that are kept too long, even at the correct temperature, can also start to deteriorate and result in food-borne illnesses.

Proper Temperatures

Your refrigerator should be set at forty degrees or colder. Your freezer should be set at zero degrees or colder. If your refrigerator or freezer does not have a temperature display inside, you can purchase an appliance thermometer at a mass retailer and check the temperatures yourself. Perishable foods should be refrigerated within two hours of preparing. If the temperature is ninety degrees or hotter, though, perishable foods need to be refrigerated within an hour.

Storage Time Guidelines

Even at the correct temperatures, there is only so long that you can store perishable food. The following table shows the maximum amounts of time that a food should be stored in a refrigerator.

▼ **HOW LONG TO REFRIGERATE FOODS**

Type of Food	Length of Time
Raw eggs	Three to five weeks
Luncheon meat (opened)	Three to five days
Luncheon meat (unopened)	Two weeks
Bacon	Seven days
Hot dogs (open package)	One week
Hamburger and ground meats	One to two days
Fresh beef, veal, lamb, and pork	Three to five days
Fresh poultry	One to two days
Leftovers	Three to four days

From the FoodSafety.gov *Storage Times for the Refrigerator and Freezer*

Frozen foods will remain safe indefinitely, though the food quality might suffer after a certain period of time. While hot dogs, luncheon meat, bacon, and sausages should ideally be eaten within one to two months of freezing, other meats can last a lot longer, with steaks retaining optimal flavor for six to twelve months in a freezer and whole chickens and turkeys lasting up to a year.

Exhaust Fans

During the normal course of cooking, there is a lot of smoke, steam, and vapors being created by the foods you are preparing. A boiling pot of pasta releases tremendous amounts of steam. Sautéing chicken in an open pan of olive oil will allow oil droppings and heat to escape into the air. Accidentally burning a piece of toast in the toaster will produce smoke that dissipates throughout the entire house. All of these elements add up and, over time, will create poor indoor air quality. The accumulation of heat and steam in the air can foster mold growth, too, causing additional health problems and structural damage to your home.

Are you having a hard time imagining how tiny bits of food and chemicals can linger in your air for so long? Consider the last time that you burned a bag of microwave popcorn or a piece of toast in the kitchen. Chances are, that distinctive burned smell did not just disappear in a matter of minutes. It probably took hours, if not days, before you could walk into the kitchen and not get a whiff. Bad smells are just an example that shows how particles that linger in the air do not disappear as fast as you might think.

When cooking, use the exhaust fan above your range only if the exhaust filters to the outside, and not simply into another portion of the house. If your fan does not exhaust to the outdoors, or if you do not have a fan, open the windows an inch or two, especially when preparing foods that might smoke or create excessive amounts of steam, and leave the window open for a brief portion of time after you are done cooking to effectively ventilate the room. Consider installing an exhaust fan in your kitchen that vents to the outside if you do not currently have one.

CHECKLIST FOR CREATING A HEALTHY KITCHEN

- ❏ Throw out nonstick cookware that has scratches and dings in the coating. Toxic chemicals can be released from a nonstick coating from high heat, but when the coating is compromised with scratches, the chemicals can be released even more.
- ❏ Use stainless steel or cast iron pots and pans instead of nonstick cookware. There are still studies being done to determine if nonstick cookware is indeed safe. Stick with time-tested basics such as stainless steel, which do not contain chemical coatings and will not release chemicals.
- ❏ Avoid plastics that could contain BPA, especially water bottles. BPA can leach out of certain plastics and contaminate your beverages with hormone-disrupting chemicals.
- ❏ Avoid letting plastics that contain PVC, such as plastic wraps, to touch your food. Chemicals can leach out of PVC plastics that are often used to directly touch your food, especially during high heat.
- ❏ Avoid polystyrene plastics, such as disposable plastics and takeout containers. Polystyrene plastics contain a carcinogen that you do not want to get into your food or drink.
- ❏ Reduce your use of plastics throughout the kitchen, and choose glass or stainless steel when possible. To be safe, use only materials that do not leach ingredients into your food or drink.
- ❏ Store foods at proper temperatures to prevent bacterial growth. It does not matter how carefully you choose your food storage items

if your food is not stored properly and becomes contaminated with pathogens.

❑ Use foods within a proper amount of time for safety reasons. Food safety starts with consuming foods during the proper time frame to avoid health problems.

❑ Use exhaust fans when cooking, especially when creating large amounts of steam. Your indoor air can become polluted with the by-products of cooking unless exhaust fans remove the particles out of your home.

CHAPTER 9

Cleaning Products

You must clean your house in order to stay healthy, right? Yes, but not the way you might think. You do not need chemicals in order to kill germs, remove grease, or clean clothes. There are plenty of natural alternatives that do the same job without the toxic exposures. But what about the kitchen and the bathroom, you might ask? Fear not, because no matter what room of the house you need to clean, there is a nontoxic alternative that will work for you.

Dangers of Household Cleaners

You are exposed to a variety of untested chemicals each day. Many of these chemicals could be ingredients in your household cleaners. While there has not been a lot of uproar about the use of untested chemicals in many other common household products, there is a growing groundswell of concern about the use of potentially hazardous chemicals used in the stuff that you clean your home with every day. That is because modern medicine is quickly learning that what you use to clean your countertops has a nasty way of ending up inside you.

ALERT

Every time the dishwasher is used, laundry is washed, or the toilet is cleaned, all of those cleaners are washed down the drain into our public waterways, where you hope that they are effectively removed before becoming part of your drinking water. For wildlife, though, there is no water filtration if these chemicals are dumped directly into their habitat, causing extensive harm.

Unregulated Products

It will probably surprise you to find out that home cleaning products have barely any regulation in the United States. The FDA does not have the jurisdiction to regulate cleaning chemicals, while the EPA only regulates products registered as pesticides, otherwise known as disinfectants.

Lack of Safety Testing

Federal law does not require any mandatory pre-market health testing for chemicals used in consumer products. It is up to the manufacturer to do the health and safety testing for the ingredients of the cleaner. Usually the testing is only done for one specific ingredient at high doses and does not account for the fact that chemicals might be mixed. For example, the health effects of mixing a carpet deodorizer with a carpet cleaner applied directly afterward are not researched, yet the chemicals could cause reactions when mixed together. Testing is done for shorter-term health effects, rather than long-term doses of the product, such as a lifetime of using a particular window cleaner.

ALERT

A majority of household cleaning products that you dispose of must be thrown away as hazardous waste. That means that you can't just simply throw them out in your weekly trash. Find out your city or municipality's hazardous waste policies and collection days and dispose of cleaners in the appropriate way.

Secret Ingredients

Under the Federal Hazardous Substances Act, manufacturers are not required to list all ingredients of household cleaners. This is so that they can protect their cleaning recipes, which are considered a trade secret. But it also means that manufacturers could put anything that they want to in your cleaner, unless it has been specifically banned by the federal government (very few chemicals are), and you will never be aware of it.

How You Are Exposed

You might assume that if you have never ingested these chemical-laden cleaners, then you should not have too much to worry about. The problem is, though, that these chemicals are getting into your body in other ways. You just don't realize it.

Sprays in the Air

A majority of liquid cleaners are designed to just spray and wipe, because it is more convenient. When you spray a liquid, though, the liquid does not just reach the surface. Tiny amounts are released into the air, too. Aerosol cans are even worse, since the spray is such a fine mist and instantly becomes a part of your indoor air. Whatever is released into the air inside your home, you will breathe in over and over again until it eventually makes its way out of your home through proper ventilation.

Residues

If you clean a surface with any type of cleaner, residues of that product are left behind. Think about what happens on a surface after you have cleaned it. Foods are placed on countertops, then ingested. A child's toy or pacifier goes right into their mouth. Pets lick carpeting and family members lie on it. Toilet bowl seats are sat upon with naked skin. Bare feet walk across newly polished floors. As you can see, household cleaners can be ingested or absorbed through your skin without you ever realizing it.

Ingestion

While the typical exposure to household cleaners is not through ingestion, it can still occur and is especially dangerous. Children and pets are at greatest risk for ingestion of cleaners. If cleaning products are not stored properly, kids can get in the bottles and drink the liquids or eat the powders. Pets can also ingest the cleaners, whether straight from the cleaning container or in a secondhand method, such as drinking toilet water that has a cleaning agent in it. Ingestion of any household cleaners is a serious danger because the quantities are greater than residual or air exposures.

Skin Exposure

Cleaning products that come in contact with the skin, whether knowingly or unknowingly, can not only cause immediate health problems on the surface of your skin, but can also be absorbed deeper into your skin and body. Using a sponge to clean a surface, your hands and arms are exposed to the cleaning materials unless you are wearing gloves. Wringing out the mop in a pail has the same effect. Bleach splashing up onto your skin while you are filling the washing machine is another example of direct skin contact.

Unhealthy Cleaners

So you might be exposed to cleaners in more ways than you had thought of. Is there any harm in that? Yes. Countless studies and research have shown that chemical-based cleaners not only cause short-term problems such as headaches and dizziness, but a whole host of other more life-threatening problems, too.

VOC Offenders

Cleaning products are one of the major sources of VOCs for homeowners, so they are also one of the easiest opportunities to rid your exposure to these unhealthy compounds. How can VOCs affect your health? VOCs can affect everyone differently, but they have been shown to cause problems such as:

- Eye, nose, and throat irritation
- Asthma
- Allergies
- Headaches
- Fatigue
- Allergic skin reaction
- Loss of coordination
- Memory impairment
- Nausea
- Liver and kidney damage
- Central nervous system damage
- Cancer

Immediate Health Effects

Direct exposure to chemical cleaning products, such as direct contact with the skin or eyes or accidentally ingesting the product, can cause immediate and sometimes fatal health effects. Those consequences are especially dire, including burns, poisoning, seizures, and death. In fact, cleaning products are the third most common source of poisoning in both adults and children.

Other immediate health problems can be caused by cleaners, too, such as skin irritation, including red, itchy skin or rashes. Many people often report feeling weak or dizzy or experiencing headaches after inhaling the fumes of cleaners. Respiratory problems, such as allergies and asthma, are another short-term health effect that can be experienced immediately following an exposure to cleaners.

DIY Solutions

Ingredients that you can find around your home make excellent cleaning solutions, and the good news is that using these ingredients are often much less expensive than buying ready-made cleaners. No chemical exposure, less health risks, and more money in your pocket. Sounds like a great solution.

FACT

Nontoxic cleaning products are often called "green cleaning" products because not only are they healthier for a human's health, but they are healthier for the environment, too. Green cleaners often derive their cleaning power from plant-derived ingredients that break down more readily in nature.

Vinegar

This versatile ingredient, which is obviously safe enough to eat, has superior cleaning power and it seems to work on just about anything around the house. You can use a small spray bottle of undiluted white vinegar to clean countertops, windows, and other durable surfaces. You can also use a half-and-half mixture of vinegar and water in a spray bottle to reduce the vinegar smell (if you do not like it), while also adding a few drops of essential oils to cover the odor.

In a demonstration by the television show *48 Hours* and *Good Housekeeping* magazine, pure white distilled vinegar was demonstrated to kill 99.9 percent of bacteria, and 90 percent of mold. Hefty cleaning power, yet still safe enough to eat.

You can easily clean your toilets with vinegar by adding a cup or two of vinegar into the toilet bowl and letting it sit for an hour or so. This can also be done overnight. Then simply scrub the toilet with a brush to clean.

Hydrogen Peroxide

You might have hydrogen peroxide in the medicine cabinet to disinfect cuts and scrapes. Well, the good news is that you can use the same hydrogen peroxide to disinfect your home, too. Hydrogen peroxide kills germs and disinfects just like bleach, yet it is safe enough to apply directly to the skin and has no foul odors that can cause health problems. The USDA has even found that hydrogen peroxide and white vinegar sanitize better than chlorine bleach.

You must be careful where you apply hydrogen peroxide, though, because it can remove color from fabrics and other surfaces just like bleach can. That is why hydrogen peroxide is great at cleaning mold and other stains in the shower and tub. Pour a small amount in a spray bottle and apply to the stain. Let sit for about an hour and come back to wipe it up. Reapply if necessary. Hydrogen peroxide can also be used to clean the toilet bowl.

ALERT

Hydrogen peroxide must be stored in an opaque bottle, such as the dark brown bottles that it is sold in. When hydrogen peroxide is exposed to sunlight for any length of time, it loses its effectiveness. Pour only the amount of hydrogen peroxide that you will need into a small spray bottle when cleaning, or attach a spray nozzle to the original bottle.

You can replace chlorine bleach, which is highly toxic to your skin and respiratory tract, with hydrogen-peroxide–based bleach, or simply use hydrogen peroxide itself. Another great aspect of hydrogen peroxide compared to chlorine bleach is that it will not contaminate waterways, since it breaks down into simple oxygen and water.

Baking Soda

This popular ingredient for cookies and other baked goods also works as a great scouring cleaner. The small white grains instantly disappear while scrubbing, yet somehow also remove stubborn, built-on dirt and grime. Mix a few tablespoons with a plant-based soap, like castile soap, for an effective scouring agent.

ESSENTIAL

To unclog a drain, try pouring one cup of baking soda down the drain, followed by one cup of white distilled vinegar. Allow to foam and fizz. Follow with a pot of hot, near boiling water poured down the drain. This process might need to be repeated often for a clogged pipe or used in conjunction with a plunger.

Tea Tree Oil

Consider adding a small bottle of tea tree oil to your cleaning routine. Tea tree oil, which can be found with other essential oils in a store, is a concentrated natural oil with a slightly medicinal smell. Tea tree oil is an antiseptic, antibacterial, and antifungal and kills mold and germs. It is safe enough to apply directly to skin and is often used in facial cleaners, but it is also an effective additive to your household cleaners. Add a few drops to a spray bottle for extra germ fighting power around the house.

Purchasing Green Cleaners

Maybe you are really not into making your own cleaners and prefer to buy something pre-made. Not a problem. It is so simple to make the change from toxic cleaners to nontoxic cleaners. Just reach for another brand of toilet bowl cleaner next time you are at the store and your job is done. You can make a dramatic impact on your family's health and the health of the planet by simply switching what you buy.

Maybe you have tried a less-harsh cleaning product in the past and it did not work very well on scrubbing the tub or cleaning your kitchen sink. There are some nontoxic cleaning products, just like conventional products, that simply are not effective. The secret is all in the formulation, just like anything else. So do not let one failed healthier cleaning attempt halt your desire to use more natural products.

Beware of Green Washing

There has been quite a movement to switch to green cleaners nationwide. It seems everyone is doing it. That also means that there are a lot of companies who are trying to profit off of this market even if they do not make truly green cleaners. Putting the picture of a green leaf or a sunny sky on a product label does not make a product nontoxic. Even the word "nontoxic" does not mean much in marketing terms, because there is no regulation for the word. It all depends on what one company's version of nontoxic might mean.

If purchasing ready-made green cleaners, choose cleaners made only from plant-derived and food-based ingredients and from companies that disclose all of their ingredients. It is not enough for a product to be made *with* a natural ingredient. A truly green cleaner is made *solely* from natural and plant-derived ingredients.

Ingredients to Avoid

There are some chemicals in cleaners that you definitely want to avoid, such as chlorine, ammonia, and lye. The problem is, though, that you can't know for sure if a cleaner even has these chemicals in them because they are not required to list the ingredients. Even if all of the ingredients were listed, there are so many that can be used in a cleaning product that it would be near impossible to have a handy list of what to avoid, and you would need a science degree to pronounce and understand them all.

Know Whom You Are Buying From

It is not fun to have to constantly read ingredient labels. It is easier to find a company whose products that you like and whose company mission mirrors your own beliefs so that you do not always have to research and investigate their products. Seventh Generation (*www.seventhgeneration.com*), Method (*www.methodhome.com*), and Ecover (*www.ecover.com/us/en/*) are examples of companies with a long-term, strong commitment toward public health and environmental concerns.

Specific Cleaning Concerns

There are always those few things at home that seem to take a lot more care and attention to keep clean. Manufacturers would like to have you believe that you need costly specialty products and equipment to take care of items such as carpets and clothing. If you get caught in this trap, though, you will be on the hook for expensive cleaners full of chemical products that are unhealthy for you and your pocketbook. There are a few nontoxic, and less costly, ways around these sticky issues.

Carpeting

Carpeting collects dust, which means plenty of allergy and asthma-inducing dust mites. Carpeting also collects allergens, mold, and bacteria that might be circulating in your home's indoor air. Combine that with the dirt and chemicals from everything that you step on every day that accumulates on the bottom of your shoes and rubs off on the carpeting's fibers, and you have got one nasty floor. If the stuff is not removed quickly, the dirt and debris gets ingrained in the fibers of carpeting. Those nasty chemicals will then migrate through the carpet into the padding below, where they will still linger but might be harder to eliminate. The cycle can be broken if you are committed to frequently cleaning your carpet before problems start to happen.

ESSENTIAL

Baking soda or cornstarch acts as a great deodorizer for the carpet. Sprinkle about one cup for an average size room lightly all over the carpet, allow it to deodorize the carpet fibers for at least thirty minutes, and then simply vacuum it up.

When you have carpeting in your home, you absolutely must own a vacuum, too. Vacuums can come with recommended cleaning agents or room deodorizers that you are told to use to keep your carpet clean and odor-free. These products are almost always full of chemicals and artificial fragrances that will simply add to the problem of poor indoor air quality, instead of helping you prevent it. Skip the use of these ingredients if possible and use chemical-free options. If your vacuum cannot be operated without a required chemical cleaning agent or deodorizer, find another vacuum that can.

The solution for heavy-duty carpet cleaning is typically steam cleaning. Steam cleaning uses water heated to high temperatures to kill dust mites and loosen grime and gunk that could be hidden in carpeting fibers. While steam cleaning is great way to remove ground-in stains and dirt, it might cause more problems than it removes. Steam cleaners, whether professional units that a technician brings to your home or home units that you can buy or rent, often require chemical cleaning solutions. Usually these cleaning agents are not exactly nontoxic. Regardless of what type of carpeting you have, it is not necessary to add even more chemicals to your carpet in the name of getting it clean. High-pressured steam should be enough to deeply clean and sanitize on its own. If you want to add something extra to boost the cleaning potential, you might be able to substitute white vinegar instead of a cleaning solution, but you should always check with the manufacturer before substituting any cleaning agents as they could cause damage to the cleaner.

ESSENTIAL

When having a professional come to your home to clean your carpets, skip the carpet deodorizer and carpet protection. These items that must be applied to your carpet are simply another source of chemicals to which your family will be exposed unnecessarily. If these items are included in the cleaning, ask if you can opt out of the services.

It is possible to remove stains from your carpeting without the need of chemical-based stain removers. Your first line of defense is to remove stains and spills on flooring as quickly as possible. Every minute that a liquid or other type of spill remains on the carpet fibers means the more that is absorbed into the carpet. You can use plain water to help remove the stain, or the fizzing action of club soda often does the trick, too. Blot the stain or spill with a clean towel until all of the residue has come up. Rinse with water, but be sure to absorb all of the moisture with a clean towel to prevent mold.

Fabric Softeners

Fabric softeners are added to a dryer or a washing machine's rinse cycle. These chemical compounds are designed to prevent static and make fabrics feel softer. The problem is that fabric softeners are designed to linger on the surface of the fabric in order to make these properties occur. That means that whatever is in the fabric softeners is directly rubbing onto your skin, whether in the clothes that you wear or the sheets and towels that you use.

While there are chemical-free liquid fabric softeners and sheets available for purchase, you can really save money and not worry about any residues by using dryer balls. Dryer balls are about the size of a tennis ball and bounce around the dryer cycle with your clothes to lift the fibers and fluff them up so that they feel soft. Dryer balls can be made of plastic, such as Nellie's dryer balls (*www.nelliesallnatural.com*), which are made with PVC-free plastic, or even just strips of wool (*www.wooldryerballs.com*), which can reduce the amount of static in your laundry because wool has natural antistatic properties. Clean, unused tennis balls can also work, too, though they are a little heavier and might be a little more rough with your clothing.

Dry-Cleaning

There are a lot of items around your home that might require dry-cleaning instead of being tossed in the washer. These items typically are made of fabrics that would be damaged by normal soap and water, or have a shape or decoration that would be damaged during a wash cycle. The care tag will say if it requires dry-cleaning or not, but your best line of defense for nontoxic cleaning is to never get an item that must be dry-cleaned in the first place.

Fabrics that are dry-cleaned are usually treated with the chemical solvent perchloroethylene, otherwise known as perc, which about 85 percent of U.S. dry cleaners still use. Perc is known to cause headaches, nausea, and dizziness and is linked to reproductive problems, as well as disorders of the central nervous system. The International Agency for Research in Cancer and the EPA have both labeled perc as a probable human carcinogen. Even worse, the chemical can stay in your body and build up in fatty tissues.

ESSENTIAL

If you must use a dry cleaner that uses perc, take your clothes out of the bag immediately after you pick them up and hang them outdoors or in a garage for at least twenty-four hours to let the fumes and chemical vapors off-gas.

There are perc-free dry cleaners, such as the Hangers Cleaners franchises, which use perc-free products. But no dry-cleaning solvent is ever going to be perfectly safe or as nontoxic as plain old soap and water. Also, you have to read between the marketing claims and find out just what the dry cleaner is using on your clothes. Beware of dry cleaners that state that they are "organic" or "natural." Chemicals are often still technically organic compounds, so question the company as to whether or not they are using perc on your clothing.

Clothing and other textiles that say that they must be dry-cleaned can often be washed in other ways, too, though it all depends on the fabric. Some items will be fine, especially if you take care to reshape them after they have been washed. Other items might actually shrink and be damaged by soap and water. If you are feeling gutsy and want to try washing an item instead of hauling it to the dry-cleaners, there are nontoxic cleaning products available that are specifically designed for delicates, such as Kooka- burra's Wool Wash (*www.kookaburraco.com*), which is made with tea tree oil and lavender.

Stain Removers

It would be nice to live in a world where spaghetti sauce is never dropped on a white shirt. Alas, we do not live in that world, so stain removers are necessary.

It is always a good idea to try a natural method to remove stains using something that you already have around the house before resorting to buying another product. For instance, cornstarch or baking soda can be used to quickly absorb fatty and oil-based stains. Sprinkle the powder on the stain, let sit for twenty minutes or more, and then brush away. If you need to treat the area again, fresh powder will work to absorb even more of the stain.

Rubbing alcohol or hairspray work to effectively remove ink stains and marker stains, whether from fabrics or from a wall. Hydrogen peroxide can work as a stain remover, too, though it can strip all color from a fabric, just like bleach. Do not dismiss the power of just simple water, whether tap water or seltzer water, at removing a stain, along with blotting the stain with an absorbent towel.

There are many natural and nontoxic stain removers available on the market that use the natural power of enzymes to break up and remove stains. You must be careful, though, that the product is as chemical-free as you would like, because most major brands now tout the power of enzymes, yet the products are anything but natural.

CHECKLIST FOR HEALTHY CLEANING

❑ Switch to cleaners that use only plant-based ingredients. Federal regulations do not require manufacturers of cleaning products to list the ingredients on the labels, so you never know what you are inhaling. Switching to 100 percent plant-based cleaners is the only way to know that you are not inhaling a toxic synthetic chemical.

❑ Look at labels and try to find out what types of chemicals are used in your cleaning products. If your cleaner does list ingredients willingly, look up the chemicals and see what the health risks are before releasing them on your surfaces and in your indoor air.

❑ Use vinegar to clean a variety of surfaces throughout your home. The same ingredient that you consume in salad dressings is highly effective at killing bacteria and mold and eliminating grime.

❑ Hydrogen peroxide is a safe and effective natural alternative to chlorine bleach. Gentle enough for medical use on your skin, yet with just as much germ-killing power as toxic bleach.

❑ Do not use harsh chemical cleaners on carpets when natural alternatives work just as well. Ditch the chemical-based cleaners the vacuum companies want you to buy at a premium and try all-natural baking soda instead.

❑ Fabric softener balls can save your family a lot of money in the long run. Eliminate laundry softeners altogether by investing in plastic or wool balls that soften fabrics for years.

❑ Avoid purchasing items that must be dry-cleaned. Clothing that must be dry-cleaned just exposes you to chemical-cleaning processes that you might want to avoid.

❑ Always air out dry-cleaned clothes before bringing them into your home. Allow the chemicals used in dry-cleaned clothes to off-gas outside before bringing them into your home to contaminate your air.

CHAPTER 10

Bathroom

If there is one room of the house where your body seems to be most intimately exposed to chemicals, it's the bathroom. Stripping down to your birthday suit to get clean, as well as the other common activities of the bathroom, leaves your body extremely vulnerable to the products and items that you use. For true healthy habits and a genuine sense of clean, a few simple changes are all it takes.

Shower Curtain

You've probably opened up a new shower curtain or shower curtain liner and noticed a distinctive smell. Many plastic and vinyl shower curtains and shower curtain liners smell a little like a new pool toy, which makes sense because they are all made from the same material—PVC.

PVC plastics can have toxic health effects throughout the home, but you are more likely to be aware of them in the bathroom when replacing a shower curtain. PVC plastic needs chemicals called plasticizers to make it soft and flexible, like a shower curtain that can bend and fold easily. These plasticizers are often made of chemicals called phthalates, which studies have shown can lead to hormonal abnormalities, thyroid disorders, birth defects, and reproductive problems. The phthalates can off-gas into your indoor air, where they are inhaled by the entire family.

Off-Gassing Chemicals

Phthalates are not the only chemicals that release from a vinyl shower curtain into your indoor air. In a 2008 study by the Center for Health, Environment & Justice and the Canadian Environmental Law Association, 108 different VOCs were released into the air after unwrapping a new shower curtain. These VOCs included such toxic chemicals such as tolulene, which is used in nail polish remover. VOCs have been linked to many health problems, ranging from eye, nose, and throat irritation, headaches, and nausea to liver damage and reproductive problems. After placing a new shower curtain in your home, you start to breathe in these compounds, some of which have been banned in some places of the world because of their health risks. The off-gassing VOCs do not just simply go away, though. In fact, the chemicals can be released into your indoor air for well over a month.

As if the phthalates and VOCs were not bad enough, there are even more substances escaping from PVC shower curtains. The study also found lead, cadmium, mercury, and chromium in vinyl shower curtains from major home retailers. Exposure to these same metals can cause massive recalls of toys and other products for children because of safety concerns, yet somehow these metals are found in the shower curtain that soaks in a kid's hot bathwater every day.

An Easy Fix

Happily, this is one of the easiest changes you can make to instantly create a healthier home. It does not cost a lot of money and it does not take a lot of time. If you do not need to replace your shower curtain or shower curtain liner, don't. Unless you have installed a new vinyl shower curtain or shower curtain liner in the past thirty days, then chances are, you do not need to make any changes, since the curtain or liner has already off-gassed much of its chemicals. If you have recently put a new vinyl shower curtain or liner in a bathroom, you will want to either dispose of it or increase the ventilation throughout your home to get the chemicals out.

When buying a new shower curtain or shower curtain liner, skip anything that says PVC or vinyl. Instead, choose a safer plastic known as PEVA or EVA plastic. PEVA or EVA plastic shower curtains have the same look and feel of vinyl shower curtains and liners, but without the toxic off-gassing of chemicals. These alternatives are widely found in major home stores and usually cost about the same as the PVC vinyl varieties. Want to go one step even better? Skip the plastic and choose a fabric shower curtain or shower curtain liner instead. Plastic, regardless of what it is, is made up of synthetic chemicals. Natural materials such as cotton are a healthier alternative.

ESSENTIAL

Plastic shower curtains can be washed to eliminate soap scrum, mold, and mildew. Place your shower curtain in the washing machine with a few dirty towels to prevent the plastic material from sticking together. Wash on the gentle cycle with cold water and detergent or hydrogen-peroxide-based bleach. Hang the curtain back up in the shower to dry.

Shower Filtration

The water coming out of your shower is the same tap water that you can drink out of your kitchen faucet. Many different chemicals, including chlorine, are added to your public drinking water supply to kill bacteria and other nasty stuff that might be lurking in the water. If you have a water filter on your tap to filter out chlorine and other materials in your drinking water, or if you will not even drink your tap water because you are concerned about what is in it, then you definitely want to consider using a filter on your showerhead. Surprisingly, your body can actually absorb more chemicals through bathing than through drinking, exposing you in a way that you might not even have thought of.

Increased Chemical Exposure

In a study conducted by the EPA, researchers found that a person has a greater exposure to the disinfecting byproducts (DBPs) in drinking water while in the shower because those chemicals can be absorbed into the skin within minutes of contact. DBPs are a health concern because they are chemicals that are formed when a disinfectant, such as chlorine, reacts with natural organic matter in any water. Just one of those DBPs produced in drinking water is chloroform, not exactly something that you want to be inhaling or absorbing through your skin. DBPs were discovered in 1974, so there has not been a lot of research on what they are, how many of them there are, or what the health effects might be.

Just the physical act of a shower makes it easier for your body to absorb whatever chemicals are in the water. Your skin is your body's largest organ, and it has been estimated that it can absorb up to 60 percent of what is put on it, including bathwater. When your skin is warm and exposed to heat, though, such as when you are in a hot shower, your pores open up, allowing more chemicals and other materials to be absorbed into your skin even more rapidly. Chemicals are more easily absorbed through the steam of a shower, too, since they vaporize easily and can become highly concentrated in the steam that is inhaled during the course of bathing.

Chlorine

Chlorine is just one of the disinfectants added to water to ensure healthy water supplies. What is so wrong with chlorine? It is a poisonous gas that is highly corrosive and very hazardous. In undiluted forms, chlorine is especially dangerous. In small amounts over long periods of time, such as in water, chlorine has health effects such as:

- Dry, brittle hair
- Dry, flaking skin
- Dandruff
- Itching
- Rashes
- Eye irritation
- Respiratory problems
- Asthma flareups

Just like swimming in a chlorinated pool for too long can cause changes in your hair and skin, bathing in highly chlorinated water day after day can cause the same problems. If you have been using countless beauty products to achieve softer hair and less irritated skin, you might want to start using a shower filter instead to potentially eliminate the source of the problem.

Of greater concern, though, is the fact that chlorine becomes chloroform when it starts to break down in water. The chloroform escapes in the steam and vapor of a hot shower, which means your chances of inhaling it are much greater than using the same source of water to wash your hands or fill a pitcher of water from the tap. Though the exposure during a shower is small, it is still a chemical exposure that can be easily prevented.

FACT

As part of the Safe Drinking Water Act, the EPA has set the maximum amount of residual chlorine that can be present in drinking water at 4 parts per million (ppm). The suggested amount of chlorine used for chlorinated pools is 1 to 4 ppm. That means your drinking water could be more heavily chlorinated than your swimming pool.

Remove the Offenders

Installing a shower filter is the only way to reduce your exposure to chemicals that are present in your water. Sure, you can also take shorter and colder showers to expose your skin to less water, and therefore less absorption, but your skin will still be regularly exposed.

Many different kinds of water filters for the shower and bath exist. For the ultimate in filtration, use a shower filter made with KDF-55, a mixture of zinc and copper alloys, which are designed to remove chlorine, heavy metals, and microbiological contaminants. KDF-55 filters work well in hot water, which, of course, is what is used in the shower. Carbon filters, however, do not work as well with hot water. Shower filters can take the place of your showerhead, or work in conjunction with your existing shower fixture. Filters are available for the tub faucet, as well, so that you do not need to fill a tub using your showerhead. Replace your filters as needed to ensure efficient chlorine and heavy metals removal.

Towels

Towels are only used against unprotected skin. Think about it. Bath towels are used on naked skin after drying off from the shower, washcloths are used on your body while in the shower, and hand towels are used to dry wet hands. You probably rub the towels briskly on your skin while bathing or drying off, increasing friction and possibly allowing residues of whatever might be hiding in the your towel's fibers to come off onto your skin. With so much direct contact between your towels and the most delicate parts of your body, why would you want to use towels with any type of toxic residue?

FACT

Most towels available on the market are made from cotton. Cotton is one of the most absorbent fibers available and can absorb seven to eight times its own weight in water. Egyptian and Pima cotton towels use a variety of cotton that has longer, stronger fibers with especially great absorption qualities.

Designer Finishes

Some towels available for purchase tout antibacterial or antimicrobial protection. These towels have been coated with a residue that is supposed to prevent bacteria from living. Sounds good in theory, doesn't it? The truth is that antibacterial finishes can actually be damaging to your health, more so than the bacteria that they are supposed to be killing. The overuse of anti-bacterial products is creating a very real problem of drug-resistant bacteria that will not respond to any prescription available because the bacteria are mutating to create "super germs." Additionally, the antibacterial coating is created out of several kinds of chemicals to adhere to the towel.

Another finish that is unnecessarily added to towels is a permanent-press finish. These finishes are designed to stop wrinkles and perhaps make the towels look like they have been freshly pressed. Permanent-press finishes have one toxic flaw: They are often created with formaldehyde. How else do you think you can preserve a flexible fabric to be wrinkle-free? Again, do you really want to use a towel on your naked skin that has a formaldehyde-based or any chemical-based residue on the fibers?

FACT

Have worn and old towels that you need to dispose of? Do not throw them in the trash, but give them new life instead. Animal shelters will take your old towels and use them as soft and warm bedding for the animals. Old towels can also be used to line pet cages, clean up messes, or dry just-bathed dogs.

Naturally Clean

Wash towels in hot water to properly kill germs and viruses that might linger. You do not need toxic antimicrobial finishes when hot water and soap will do the same thing. Allow towels to dry out after using them by hanging them on a hook or towel bar to prevent the formation of bacteria and mold. If you have recently bought a new set of towels and are concerned about chemical residues but do not want to replace the towels, wash the towels in hot water and detergent several times and hang them out in the hot sun to dry. While many finishes will not completely be removed from a towel no matter how many times you wash it, you can dramatically reduce the amount of chemical product left behind with lots of hot water and exposure to the hot sun.

If possible, do not replace your towels simply because you have changed the color scheme of your room. Older towels will have a lot of the harmful chemicals and dyes washed out by now, so they might be a healthier alternative than buying new products. When browsing the store aisles to replace your worn towels, avoid any type of artificial finish, such as an antimicrobial coating or a nonwrinkle finish. Marketing claims such as "kills germs," "prevents germs," "won't wrinkle," and "wrinkle-free" are indications that a towel might have been chemically treated with a finish.

ESSENTIAL

For the ultimate in chemical-free products, choose organic cotton or bamboo towels. Organic cotton and bamboo are grown without the use of harmful pesticides. Just because a towel is made from organic cotton or bamboo does not mean that it is necessarily chemical-free, though. Look for products that are also made with nontoxic dyes or unbleached.

Toilet Paper

Toilet paper is used on some of the most sensitive and delicate parts of your body. Softness can be a real concern for products used in this area. While you do not want to be using a product that feels like sandpaper, you might find that you do not need the fancy ultra-plush toilet papers, wipes, and other products designed for sensitive skin if your private areas are not being irritated from chemical-laden toilet papers that you might use each day.

FACT

Americans spend more than six billion dollars on toilet paper each year, more than any other country in the world. On average, people in the United States use fifty-seven squares each day. That averages out to about fifty pounds of toilet paper used by each person each year.

Toilet paper is often whitened and bleached with chlorine. There are ways to achieve white toilet paper using totally chlorine-free (TCF) or processed chlorine-free (PCF) techniques, and many manufacturers use them.

Other chemicals used in producing toilet paper can be inks, dyes, and perfumes. Some brands add lotion for added comfort while other options include pre-moistened wipes that entirely eliminate the dry toilet paper option. All of these additives have to be made of something, and usually they are chemicals that you might not want to expose the very sensitive parts of your body to on a daily and intimate basis.

When choosing a toilet paper, look for one that states that it is free of inks, dyes, and perfumes. Toilet paper made with TCF or PCF techniques are good choices, too. If you experience sensitivity, swelling, or redness, consider using another brand of toilet paper to see if that is the cause.

Bath Mats

Bath mats have the same health risks as towels do. The cushiony mat that is under your wet feet straight out of the shower is in direct contact with your skin. If the mat is coated with unnecessary chemical finishes, though, those residues can potentially rub off onto your skin. Antibacterial and permanent-press finishes are common among bath mats, as are mold-killing finishes. The finishes might all be made of different ingredients, but there is a common truth among them—they are unnecessary if you simply clean your bath mats as you should.

ESSENTIAL

Bath mats can be a safety hazard when they do not stay securely in place on the bathroom floor. Prevent accidental slips and falls by purchasing bath mats with a nonslip backing. Bath mats can also be made safer with self-adhesive strips of nonslip materials applied to the underside of the mat.

Bath mats should be washed in hot water with detergent frequently to kill germs and mold. If you have a bath mat that cannot be put in the wash, such as a sisal rug, place it outside in full sun frequently to let the power of nature disinfect the item from germs. Periodically check the underside of your bath mat for any sign of mold growth. If there is mold, that might indicate a larger moisture problem in your bathroom.

Medicine Cabinet

Regardless of what types of products that you have in your medicine cabinet, they can become a health hazard if not taken care of properly or if kept for too long. Medicine cabinets are often located in a bathroom, the one place of the house where your medicine should not be. The hot, humid, and wet conditions of a bathroom are not good for medications and can cause them to break down. If possible, you want to store medications in a cool, dry place, such as in another room or in a closet. If you have children in the house, always purchase medications in childproof containers and keep them out of the reach of children and pets.

Expiration Dates

Expiration dates of medications pose another potential health hazard, as well. You might forget how much time has passed since you bought a box of allergy medicine, and the expiration date might have already come and gone. At least twice a year, go through your entire medicine cabinet and dispose of anything that is past the listed expiration date. Look at all of the products that you might have, from pain relievers and ointments to eye drops and contact lens solution. Keep medications in their original packaging, which will have the expiration date clearly listed. If you transfer pills or other products into a pill box or another container, you will not know the expiration date.

When to Toss Cosmetics

Other items in your bathroom, such as shampoo and moisturizers, might not necessarily have expiration dates, but should be used in a certain time frame, as well, for optimal safety. There is no law for cosmetics to have expiration dates. Does that mean that you would want to use a tube of mascara that is five years old, though? Probably not. While preservatives found in cosmetic items might keep bacteria under check for a while, they will not last forever. If you strive to use items that are as natural and preservative-free as possible, those products will likely diminish even faster.

Policing your cosmetics and body care products to make sure that they are still safe to use is entirely up to you. The following are time frames after which you should toss the product just to be sure:

▼ **WHEN TO TOSS COSMETICS**

Cosmetic	Shelf Life
Liquid foundation	Three to six months
Concealer	Six to eight months
Powders (pressed powder, eye shadow, blush)	One year
Mascara	Three months
Lip gloss and lipstick	One year
Eye and lip pencils	One year
Facial cleansers and moisturizers	Six months
Facial toners	One year
Natural cosmetics and body care products	Six months

If you tend to hold on to products for quite a while before using them up, consider writing the date that you started using the product on the label so that you will know how long it has been opened.

Regardless of how new or old your cosmetics are, they can still harbor bacteria if your brushes are not clean. Synthetic brushes should be washed once a week, while natural bristle brushes should be washed once a month using a mild soap or baby shampoo. Disposable sponges should be used only once and washed before reuse.

CHECKLIST FOR A HEALTHY BATHROOM

❑ Do not purchase vinyl or PVC shower curtains or liners. One of the biggest sources of indoor air pollution in your bathroom is the vinyl shower curtain, which can release more than 100 pollutants. PVC-free shower liners are easily available and do not cost much more than vinyl ones.

❑ Use a shower filter. Just like your tap water, your shower water can contain pollutants that you might not want to expose your body to, especially in the steam of a hot shower. Filter your shower water just like your tap water.

❑ Avoid towels with antimicrobial or permanent press finishes. Don't wipe off with a towel only to be exposed to residues of germ-killing chemicals or formaldehyde resins.

❏ Use PEVA or EVA plastic shower curtains and liners, or ones made of cloth. Avoid the problems with vinyl shower curtains by choosing a less-toxic plastic or a fabric alternative.

❏ Check your bath mat periodically for mold growth. Black spots underneath your bath mat can be mold, which rapidly accumulates on this item that is often left damp.

❏ Use toilet paper with as few additives as possible. Prevent skin reactions to chemical additives by choosing toilet paper that is as unaltered as possible.

❏ Periodically check your medicine cabinet for expired products. It is often easy to forget how much time has gone by since you purchased a product, but expired products can lose their effectiveness or be unsafe.

❏ Toss cosmetic items that have been opened for longer than the suggested "use by" time frames. Bacterial growth can occur in products after a certain time frame, when the preservatives in the item are no longer effective.

CHAPTER 11

Killing Germs

If you listen to television commercials, watch the news, or flip through a magazine, then you might be on the verge of becoming a germaphobe—someone who is obsessed with cleanliness and killing bacteria. There is nothing wrong with making sure that things are clean, but the national obsession with how and where we kill germs seems to be getting a little off track. Some germs are necessary and good, and you certainly do not need an arsenal of synthetic chemical products to kill the ones that are bad.

Not All Germs Are Bad

The word "germ" tends to have a very negative image today, but in truth, germs can actually be healthy and beneficial. Of course you want to kill the bad germs, but in doing so, it will be extremely beneficial to you to let the good ones survive.

What Are Germs?

Germs are tiny living organisms that can cause disease. Germs do not just affect humans; they can affect plants and animals, too. These organisms are typically classified in four different categories:

- **Bacteria.** These one-celled organisms feed off of the surroundings in their environment and can cause infections, such as strep throat and cavities. But not all bacteria are bad, and the bacteria in your gut are highly beneficial.
- **Viruses.** If a virus is not located inside a living cell, called a host, it cannot live for very long. If a virus does get into your body, though, it can reproduce and cause illnesses such as the flu and chicken pox.
- **Fungi.** Made up of many cells and feeding off of humans, fungi like to live in damp, warm places, and are the cause of conditions such as athlete's foot.
- **Protozoa.** Typically found in water, these one-celled organisms can cause intestinal problems such as cramps, diarrhea, and nausea.

Beneficial Bacteria

There are 100 trillion bacterial cells in your body right now—ten times the number of human cells that are in your body. Bacteria are thriving on your skin and in your gut, rapidly multiplying before quickly dying off, but do not worry. These bacteria are something that you want to have.

Your gut, which includes your small and large intestines and colon, is home to trillions of beneficial bacteria. These bacteria are the very things that help you digest your food. Without good bacteria, you would not be able to break down plant starches. In fact, the amount of bacteria that are in your gut could be linked to your risk for obesity, according to researchers such as Ruth Ley at Cornell University's Department of Microbiology. If your body is unable to process foods because of a lack of good bacteria, it could possibly lead to weight gain and obesity, among other diseases.

Bacteria thrive on your skin, too, where they create an invisible barrier to protect your body from harmful elements. Dr. Julia Segre, with the National Human Genome Research Institute, found that in the crook of your elbow, there are a variety of different types of bacteria that moisturize the skin by digesting the fats that your skin produces. Even if you wash this area of your skin, more than one million bacteria will still exist in each square centimeter of the crook of your elbow. By digesting naturally occurring skin fats, bacteria on all areas of your skin help protect your skin from chapping and cracking, which would allow harmful germs to enter and take hold.

FACT

The National Institute of Health's Common Fund has started the Human Microbiome Project (*https://commonfund.nih.gov/hmp*) to study the germs, including beneficial bacteria, that are commonly found in nasal passages, oral cavities, the skin, gastrointestinal tract, and urogenital tract and understand how they affect our health and whether they can be altered to help fight disease.

Increasing Your Bacteria

Both on your skin and in your gut, the more beneficial bacteria there are, the less room there is for bad bacteria to come in and multiply. So how can you increase the amount of good bacteria in your system? It all depends on what you eat and the supplements you might take.

Probiotics and prebiotics can help stimulate the growth of beneficial bacteria in your body. While probiotics are the actual living organisms, prebiotics are just nondigestible foods that aid in the growth of bacteria. Both probiotics and prebiotics can be added to foods that tout the claims of increasing your beneficial gut bacteria, such as certain yogurt brands or drinks. Probiotics can also be sold in a supplement form, such as in a capsule or a powder.

You do not need to buy specialty foods with marketing claims, though, in order to increase your healthy bacteria levels. You just need to eat the right types of foods. Probiotics can be naturally found in foods such as:

- Yogurt
- Miso
- Tempeh
- Fermented and unfermented milk

Prebiotics, because they are undigestible food ingredients, are typically found in high fiber foods, such as:

- Wheat and whole grains, including oatmeal
- Onions
- Garlic
- Leeks
- Greens, such as chard and kale
- Artichokes
- Bananas
- Flax
- Barley
- Legumes

Limit Antibiotics

Your body is filled with beneficial bacteria that it needs to survive and thrive. Every time you take an antibiotic, though, both the bad bacteria and good bacteria are killed off, altering your chemical makeup. While sometimes it is necessary to take an antibiotic, many times antibiotics are prescribed when they are not necessary because patients demand them and doctors relent and write prescriptions for them.

Antibiotics are necessary for bacterial infections, such as strep throat, urinary tract infections, wound and skin infections, some ear infections, and severe sinus infections. Typically, the only true way to know if an infection is caused by bacteria is to take a test, such as a throat culture.

Viral infections, which are caused by viruses and not bacteria, will not respond to antibiotic use. Viral infections can include the flu, most coughs, most ear infections, colds, most sore throats, bronchitis, and stomach flu. The American College of Physicians estimates that more than 133 million courses of antibiotics are prescribed to patients in nonhospital settings each year, yet up to 50 percent of those prescriptions are thought to be unnecessary because they are given for viral infections. If you are sick and visit a doctor who wants to give you a prescription, ask if an antibiotic is necessary and discuss your concerns with her.

Antibacterials

Germs, which include bacteria, exist everywhere. That is a fact of life that we must come to terms with. Do we need to kill germs? Yes, sometimes, but there are more natural and safer ways to do it without exposing yourself to antibacterial chemicals whose long-term health effects are still not known and are now under intense scrutiny.

Triclosan

How do we suddenly have products that can kill germs where germ-killing power never existed before? A powerful antibacterial chemical called triclosan was let loose from its original hospital setting, and now the world seems to be hooked.

Triclosan is a broad-spectrum antimicrobial agent that kills bacteria, fungi, and mildew. Triclosan is registered as a pesticide with the EPA, because it kills living things, which in this case are microorganisms. When triclosan is used in personal care products, though, the same chemical is not considered a pesticide due to federal laws. Triclosan is used in toothpaste, soaps, and other personal care products that are regulated by the FDA.

Hand sanitizers, antibacterial toothpastes, and bacteria-killing socks, many of which use triclosan, are a modern-day invention of just the past generation or two. Antibacterial agents have made their way into almost every aspect of everyday life, but that might not be a good thing because there are scientific studies raising concerns over whether triclosan can interfere with the endocrine system, start interfering with hormones, and create problems far, far worse than a couple of days of the sniffles. There are other concerns with triclosan, too, such as the formation of drug-resistant bacteria, which means that bacteria that cause colds and sore throats and other serious health problems will not respond to the medicines that we have to treat those conditions.

ALERT

Even though the concerns about triclosan and its possible health effects on the endocrine system are becoming more widely known, the EPA is not scheduled to conduct another comprehensive review of the chemical again until the year 2013. This review will actually occur ten years earlier than originally planned because of the increasing amounts of scientific evidence coming in.

Before you start thinking that exposure to triclosan is not a concern for you, consider these surprising facts. Seventy-five percent of the U.S. population has triclosan in their urine. The chemical has also been found in 97 percent of tested breast milk.

Overuse in Society

Synthetic antibacterial agents are not just used in hand sanitizers and personal care products. They can also be found in a shocking array of consumer goods that you would not even think about, including:

- Paints
- Flooring
- Food storage
- School supplies
- Sinks
- Countertops
- Refrigerators
- Toilets
- Vacuums
- Air purifiers

Though it is important to prevent the transmission of bad germs, you might not be comfortable your family's exposure to items embedded with a chemical still under research for health and safety. Always read the labels of everything that you buy. If the product touts antimicrobial protection, such as stating that it uses the trademarks of Microban or Biofresh, you will want to weigh the pros and cons of your exposure to the antibacterial product.

How to Avoid Triclosan

Go through your cabinets and look for any products that might contain triclosan. Antibacterial soaps, body washes, and toothpastes are all considered over-the-counter drugs, so if triclosan is contained in those ingredients, it must be listed on the label, by law. Cosmetics containing triclosan must list the ingredient on the product label, as well.

If you want to avoid triclosan exposure in any product that you use, you must be vigilant about reading labels and marketing claims. While triclosan must be listed as an ingredient on over-the-counter drugs and cosmetics, it can occur in many other products in the home without being listed as an ingredient. If a product that you buy says that it is antibacterial, antimicrobial, fights odors, or kills germs, you might want to investigate exactly how it does that, whether by natural means or, more likely, an antibacterial chemical. Even products that are not labeled as antibacterial, though, such as shaving gel, can contain triclosan.

FACT

Triclosan is now very present in our public waterways. The U.S. Geological Survey found triclosan in 58 percent of the rivers and streams that it tested. Bacteria are part of the way that nature works, yet waterways now contain a chemical that is designed to kill bacteria, potentially disrupting the normal ebb and flow of nature.

Surprisingly, dish detergents can contain triclosan, so read the labels or contact the company to find out if the detergent contains this ingredient. Kitchen sponges often contain antimicrobial properties, as well. Many of the sponges available today claim antibacterial properties, so look for pure cellulose sponges that have no chemical additives. Want to naturally kill the germs that breed in sponges? Wet the sponge and then microwave it for two minutes to kill the germs without the need of chemicals, or put it in the top rack of your dishwasher with every load.

Hand Sanitizers versus Hand Washing

Flashy marketing campaigns would have you believe that you can't kill germs unless you use an antibacterial product. Nowadays, there is a hand-sanitizer dispenser at the grocery store, the department store, on cruise ships, at banks, and anywhere else that people congregate. The proliferation of hand sanitizing products found everywhere could lead you to believe that they are superior in killing germs, but medical research tells another story.

Doctors Weigh In

Amidst all of the potential health concerns of triclosan and debates on whether or not it is even necessary or safe in our daily lives, there have been some big name players in the field of health and safety that have come forward saying that the use of the chemical is not even necessary in the fight against germs. Many more studies have proven that good old-fashioned soap and water work just as well as triclosan-containing products.

ESSENTIAL

You can control the spread of germs by not touching your eyes, mouth, or nose before washing your hands. Viruses and bacteria from another person's cough or sneeze can live from twenty minutes to more than two hours on surfaces such as doorknobs and tables.

The American Medical Association's "Use of Antimicrobial Agents in Consumer Products" report stated "there is little evidence to support the use of antimicrobials in consumer products such as topical hand lotions and soaps." The report went on to say "it is prudent to avoid the use of antimicrobial agents in consumer products."

The FDA's "Triclosan: What Consumers Should Know" (*www.fda.gov/forconsumers/consumerupdates/ucm205999.htm*) states that "the agency does not have evidence that triclosan in antibacterial soaps and body washes provides any benefit over washing with regular soap and water."

Even the Centers for Disease Control (CDC), in the midst of the 2009 H1N1 flu epidemic, stated that the best technique for washing your hands to avoid getting the flu was to use soap and warm water for fifteen to twenty seconds. The CDC suggested alcohol-based wipes or gel sanitizers only when soap and water were not available.

Proper Hand Washing

How many people do you know that have a bottle of hand sanitizer right by their kitchen sink and will use that product before they use soap and water, thinking that they are receiving superior germ fighting power? Unfortunately, they have been led to believe that they will be healthier by relying on a chemically made sanitizer, but they could be wrong.

The CDC's "Handwashing: Clean Hands Saves Lives" (*www.cdc.gov/handwashing*) says that "washing hands with soap and water is the best way to reduce the number of germs on them" and that "sanitizers do not eliminate all types of germs." To effectively kill as many germs on your hands as possible, follow the CDC's recommended steps to wash your hands:

1. Wet your hands with clean, running water (warm or cold) and apply soap.
2. Rub your hands together to make a lather and scrub them well; be sure to scrub the backs of your hands, between your fingers, and under your nails.
3. Continue rubbing your hands for at least twenty seconds. Need a timer? Hum the "Happy Birthday" song from beginning to end twice.
4. Rinse your hands well under running water.
5. Dry your hands using a clean towel or air-dry them.

When washing your hands with soap and water to avoid the use of triclosan, make sure that your hand soap does not contain the chemical, either. In a study by the EWG, 43 percent of hand soaps contained triclosan.

Hand Sanitizers

Sometimes you just cannot get access to running water and soap, such as when you are on a mountain hike, on an excursion, or in an emergency. In those cases, hand sanitizers can be handy to reduce the amount of germs that are on your hands. The CDC recommends that if soap and water are not available, use an alcohol-based sanitizer that contains at least 60 percent alcohol. However, the CDC warns that "hand sanitizers are not effective when hands are visibly dirty."

There are hand sanitizers that kill germs using natural ingredients instead of the harsh chemicals and synthetic fragrances often found in conventional hand sanitizers. CleanWell (*www.cleanwelltoday.com*), Burt's Bees (*www.burtsbees.com*), and JASON (*www.jason-natural.com*) are among the companies that have natural germ-killing brands.

Disinfectants

Keeping your hands clean is important, but you might also want a product to keep the other surfaces in your house germ-free, as well, especially if someone in your home has a cold or flu. Disinfectant sprays are a great way to effectively kill germs on hard surfaces when the need arises.

Registered Pesticides

Disinfectants are designed to kill living things. In this case, the living things are microorganisms such as viruses and bacteria. Any product that is considered a disinfectant must be registered with the EPA. When a disinfectant product makes a claim that it kills 99.9 percent of germs, that claim must be verified by the EPA. In fact, you should look for an EPA registration number on the label of any disinfectant to make sure that it has been tested. If there is an EPA registration number, then you know that all of the wording on the product label has been reviewed and approved. Manufacturers are required to submit testing data on the effectiveness of their product as part of the registration for the disinfectant. Regardless of what ingredients are used in a disinfectant, whether they are chemical or natural, the product still must be verified and regulated by the EPA.

Commercially Prepared Disinfectants

You might be familiar with chemical based disinfectants that proudly claim that they kill 99.9 percent of viruses and bacteria. These products will kill the germs that you want to get rid of. However, did you know that you can use plant-based ingredients to kill the same amount of germs, too, without exposing yourself to chemicals?

Though plant-based disinfectants were largely unheard of just a few years ago, they are now readily available and are proven to kill germs. Companies such as Seventh Generation (*www.seventhgeneration.com*) and Method (*www.methodhome.com*) have disinfectant products that utilize the natural germ fighting power of CleanWell (*www.cleanwelltoday.com*). CleanWell, a patented formula that uses thyme oil, was created by a father whose son was born with a severe immune deficiency condition. Benefect (*www.benefect .com*) also uses the power of thyme to create a botanically based disinfectant.

Common Household Disinfectants

You do not need to buy a specialty product for disinfecting power when many items that you might already have at home will work, too. Vinegar can kill germs, as well as mold. Hydrogen peroxide works on killing germs, too, and is designed for human exposure. When you combine the power of vinegar and hydrogen peroxide together, though, they work as an extremely effective germ killer. By spraying a surface first with white vinegar, then with 3 percent hydrogen peroxide, the liquids combine to make peracetic acid, which kills germs such as *Salmonella* and *E. coli* bacteria. Do not mix the two liquids together in one bottle, though, because it can be dangerous.

Bleach is also an effective disinfectant, though you do need to take proper precautions when using it. Hydrogen peroxide–based bleach is preferable to chlorine-based bleach. When using bleach as a germ killer, combine one part bleach with four parts water.

Steam Cleaning

In the quest to kill germs throughout your home, water might be all that you need to sanitize and disinfect surfaces. When water is heated and creates steam, the hot temperatures and water vapor can kill germs naturally. There are many different products that are available for use in the home to clean and disinfect using the power of steam. Shark (*www.sharkclean.com*), Hoover (*www.hoover.com*), and Bissell (*www.bissell.com*) offer mops and vacuums that use steam to clean floors, as well as portable steam cleaners that can be used in places such as the tub and on countertops. In order to clean and disinfect naturally, it is important not to use chemical cleaning agents with the steam cleaners, just the steam alone.

There are products that also use the power of steam to clean and sterilize baby bottles, such as those from Tommee Tippee (*www.tommeetippee.us*), Nuk (*www.nuk.com*), Philips Avent (*www.avent.com*), and Bebek (*www.bebekbabyproducts.com/usa*). Germ Terminator (*www.germterminator.com*) offers a steam-powered toothbrush sterilizer. Guardian Technologies (*www.guardiantechnologies.com*) even offers a toothbrush sanitizer and nursery sanitizer that use the germ-killing power of dry heat, without any water at all, to kill microorganisms.

CHECKLIST FOR KILLING GERMS

- ❑ Realize that not all germs are bad and you cannot kill them all. Your body cannot properly prepare itself to fight off germs if it is never given a chance, and some germs are actually necessary for good health. Find a balance in the way that you prevent the spread of germs from someone with a cold and in trying to rid your entire home and body from common everyday germs.
- ❑ Avoid the use of triclosan in your home. Constantly relying on the severe germ-killing power of this drug can reduce the effectiveness of germ killers when you really need them. Triclosan is also being investigated for other health concerns that are far worse than the common cold.
- ❑ Wash hands with soap and water for the most effective germ killing. Simple, old-fashioned soap and water still is the most effective way to kill germs and is recommended by major medical agencies.
- ❑ Use hand sanitizers only when soap and water are not available. These alcohol-based cleaners should be used only when soap and water cannot be found.

❑ Avoid touching your mouth, eyes, and nose with your hands to prevent the spread of germs. Reduce the way that germs are spread and they won't.

❑ Plant-based disinfectants can effectively kill germs. All disinfectants must pass the same EPA guidelines, so whether they are made from chemicals or natural ingredients, they work just as effectively.

❑ Hydrogen peroxide, vinegar, and hydrogen peroxide–based bleach can kill germs using products you already have around the house. Kill germs more naturally, and without as much expense, using common household ingredients and not specialty cleaners.

❑ Steam cleaning kills microorganisms using just highly heated water. Forget the use of any cleaners and just use hot water instead.

CHAPTER 12

Personal Care Products and Cosmetics

The traditional beauty industry has a very ugly side to it. It is a tale of toxic ingredients, questionable marketing practices, legal loopholes, and lack of safety testing. Though consumers put faith in the safety of the products that they apply to their bodies each day, that faith is often unwarranted. There is a happy ending, though. You can have thick, shiny hair, an acne-free complexion, and glowing skin without being a human guinea pig for little understood cosmetic ingredients. You simply need to know where to look.

Shocking Truths about Cosmetic Regulations

When you go into a store to pick up some deodorant, a new tube of lipstick, and some sunscreen for your child, you probably do not think much about what you are buying, beside the name brand and how much it costs. After all, you probably assume that if something is being sold on the shelves of your favorite store, it has been tested to be healthy and safe, right? Think again.

Cosmetics Defined

It does not matter if you are a man, woman, or child. You are using cosmetics, at least in the way that the FDA defines them. A cosmetic is defined as "articles intended to be rubbed, poured, sprinkled, or sprayed on, introduced into, or otherwise applied to the human body." This is a big deal, because cosmetic safety regulations do not just affect anyone who wears makeup; they affect your entire family. If you practice any semblance of health and hygiene, from using soap in the shower to brushing your teeth, you are exposed to a variety of cosmetics each and every day.

Federal Food, Drug, and Cosmetic Act

Shocking but true: The cosmetics industry is largely unregulated. All of the lotions and potions that you put on your skin and around your eyes and on your lips and nails are not necessarily tested by the government for health and human safety. Surprising, isn't it? "But how can that be?" you might ask. That is a very good question.

The FDA does not have the legal authority over the cosmetics industry that you might think. According to the FDA's Office of Cosmetics and Colors, "Under the Federal Food, Drug, and Cosmetic Act, cosmetic products and ingredients do not require FDA approval before they go on the market. The exception is color additives (other than those used in most hair dyes). Companies and individuals who market cosmetics have the legal responsibility to ensure the safety of their products."

Lack of Health and Safety Testing

Even more shocking, cosmetic products do not even have to do any safety testing. According to the FDA, "Failure to adequately substantiate the safety of a cosmetic product or its ingredients prior to marketing causes the product to be misbranded unless the following warning statement appears conspicuously on the principal display panel of the product's label: 'Warning—The safety of this product has not been determined.'" Do you read all of the warnings and information on the back of the package of each and every cosmetic item that you buy?

Regardless of whether safety testing has been done or not, the testing still rests in the hands of the cosmetic industry professionals, not a third-party regulatory agency. A Cosmetic Industry Review (CIR) panel is in charge of the determination of health and safety of the products that you use each day. The FDA states "The CIR is an independent, industry-funded panel of medical and scientific experts that meets quarterly to assess the safety of cosmetic ingredients. The limitations are that the CIR bases its reviews on summaries provided by the manufacturers, not the complete data sets from safety testing, and reviews only a limited selection of ingredients each year. FDA may or may not agree with CIR conclusions."

FACT

Have you had a negative reaction to a cosmetic product? The FDA wants to know about it. Report your problem to the FDA (*www.fda.gov/ForConsumers/ConsumerUpdates/ucm241820.htm*). According to Linda Katz, MD, director of the FDA's Office of Cosmetics and Colors, "Consumers are one of FDA's most important resources when it comes to identifying problems."

So, all of the products that you use on your skin—up to 60 percent of which can be absorbed into your body, by the way—are not tested by the government and it is up to the people who sell them to do all of the health and human safety testing. The people who stand to make millions, if not billions, of dollars from selling you something are the very ones who are supposed to tell you whether or not it is safe.

The FDA cannot even act on a cosmetic until it has been put on the market, and then only when it has been established that the product is harmful to consumers. Even then, the FDA is limited by time and resources. According to the FDA, cosmetic firms "are not legally required to tell FDA about their products and safety data," and the "FDA does not have the resources to sample and analyze all cosmetics on the market." The FDA does not even have the authority to issue a recall for harmful cosmetics.

Banned Ingredients

With thousands of chemicals used in cosmetics, though, just a handful have actually been limited or banned in cosmetics, including:

- Bithionol
- Mercury compounds
- Vinyl chloride in aerosol products
- Halogenated salicylanilides
- Zirconium in aerosol products
- Chloroform
- Methylene chloride
- Chlorofluorocarbons
- Prohibited cattle materials

There are many well-known potentially harmful ingredients that still have not made the restricted list yet, such as lead. Even though the health hazards of lead are well documented, a study by the Campaign for Safe Cosmetics found lead in 61 percent of lipsticks that it tested. The FDA tested those lipsticks, as well, following the Campaign for Safe Cosmetics study and also found lead, which it detailed in "Lipstick and Lead: Questions and Answers" (*www.fda.gov/cosmetics/productandingredientsafety/productinformation/ucm137224.htm*). Though lead is a known neurotoxin, it is legal to have it in cosmetics that are applied to your skin and that might be ingested.

Avoiding Unhealthy Ingredients

With so many chemicals in use in so many different products, many of which have never been adequately tested for health and human safety, it is difficult to simply say "avoid these ingredients" because there are too many to name. It is also challenging to clearly state what the health consequences of all of these synthetic chemicals might be because they are all so varied and they are still being tested. Health effects can range from rashes to cancer, with the more serious health risks coming from long-term exposure.

Skin Deep Cosmetics Database

There are thousands of chemicals in use in cosmetics. There are also hundreds of brands with different products and formulations that seem to change several times throughout the year. Every few months there is a new, improved conditioner for sale or a revolutionary lipstick with benefits that have never been achieved before. How can you stay up-to-date with the health and safety issues of products that you apply to your body when you have got so much else to do in life, too?

The Environmental Working Group's (EWG) Skin Deep Cosmetics Database (*www.ewg.org/skindeep*) is the answer for consumers who are concerned about their cosmetics safety and want to find unbiased information that is easily available. Started in 2004, the Skin Deep Cosmetics Database offers consumers safety profiles of specific ingredients and even specific products by brand name so that you can make an informed choice. The EWG states that "Our aim is to fill in where industry and government leave off."

EWG has scientists who research ingredients used in cosmetics in the United States and then compares those ingredients with nearly sixty databases of regulated and toxic substances to create a safety snapshot of a particular ingredient or product. More than 69,000 products and more than 2,800 brands are referenced on the website.

FACT

The EWG is a founding member of the Campaign for Safe Cosmetics (*www.safecosmetics.org*), a coalition of health, environmental, and consumer groups. The Campaign for Safe Cosmetics actively strives to educate consumers about health dangers in cosmetics and encourage the health and beauty industry to use safer ingredients in cosmetics.

When you enter a specific product name in the search engine of the Skin Deep Cosmetics Database, you will receive easy-to-understand graphics of how healthy or unsafe that product is. A chart that lists the health concerns of ingredients ranks the risks of hazards such as cancer or allergies from low to high. The list of ingredients is posted, and each ingredient is given a hazard score from zero to ten, with zero being the safest and ten having high risks. When researching specific ingredients, you can find out what the ingredient is used for as well as all of the health hazards based on specific toxicity reports.

Common Ingredients to Avoid

Even though there are thousands of chemicals used in cosmetics, there are a few that stand out as ones to avoid. The EWG lists the following common ingredients as ones with safety concerns, including the presence of harmful contaminants:

- Fragrance
- DMDM hydantoin
- Diazolidinyl urea
- Imidazolidinyl urea
- Ceteareth
- Polyethylene glycol and PEG

There are many, many more ingredients that also have health hazards, though, such as parabens, oxybenzone, phthalates, retinyl palmitate, hydroquinone, and others. EWG's "Top Tips for Safer Products" (*www.ewg.org/skindeep/top-tips-for-safer-products/#pick_safer*) offers a lengthier list broken down into ingredients to avoid in specific categories, as well as ingredients to avoid for men, women, and children.

Of course it is not always easy to remember these strange chemical names, especially when you might not even be able to pronounce them, much less spell them. You can write down the list of common health hazards found in cosmetics and keep it with you while shopping. The EWG also offers a pocket guide, "Quick Tips for Safer Cosmetics," with a $5 donation so that you can put it in your purse or wallet and access all of the information that you need when shopping for cosmetics.

Label Claims

To avoid potentially unhealthy ingredients, you need to read the labels. Reading the labels is the only way that you have to know what is in a product, but those labels can often be very misleading. It can be difficult to wade through the marketing claims to really discover what is in a product.

Misleading Marketing

There is very little regulation with labeling terms on cosmetics. The words "hypoallergenic" and "natural" mean nothing, at least legally. There is no government standard or benchmark that must be met to allow a product to use these terms. Just because a product has a picture of a leaf or a cucumber slice on the packaging does not mean that it is made primarily from all natural ingredients. It might have one or two natural ingredients, if at all, and the rest are all synthetic.

Even the term "fragrance-free" does not legally have to mean what you think it means. The term "fragrance-free" can simply mean the product has no smell, not that fragrances were not added. Often, there are many synthetic fragrances in the product just masking each other.

FACT

"Pinkwashing" is the term when companies who want to boost profits associate their products with the fight against breast cancer, when in actuality ingredients in those products are linked to causing breast cancer. While there are many companies who truly are committed to the fight against breast cancer, it is important to support those that do not use cancer-causing ingredients.

Organic Certifications

The term "organic" is regulated by the U.S. Department of Agriculture (USDA), but only with food ingredients. So if you are looking for a "100 percent organic" cosmetic, with a USDA Organic seal, then the product is only going to contain food ingredients, such as oils and spices.

Cosmetics can be labeled "Organic" and carry the USDA Organic seal if they contain at least 95 percent organically produced food ingredients. Next best is the term "Made with Organic Ingredients," which means the cosmetic won't carry the USDA Organic seal, but the product must still contain at least 70 percent organically produced food ingredients.

Seals of Approval and Certifications

Do not be fooled by fancy-looking certification seals on cosmetics. There are many European certifications such as EcoCert (*www.ecocert .com*), IOS Natural and Organic Cosmetic Standard (*www.certechregistration .com/1_organic_certification.htm*), and BDIH Certified Natural Cosmetics (*www.kontrollierte-naturkosmetik.de/e/index_e.htm*), which do mean that a cosmetic item has been held to strict organic and all natural standards. But you might find some other seals of "certification" that do not mean much. If you are buying a product based on a certification, check it out and see what the certifying standards are. Any brand or organization can come up with a seal or certification claim, so it is up to you to see what the claim means and how it was tested.

Cleaning Up Your Cosmetics

You might be scared to use anything in your shower or medicine cabinet right now after learning about the near-lack of regulation for the many items that you use on your body. It is important not to stress too much, though. The good news is that now that you know what the problems are, you have the power to fix them.

Investigate Your Products

Look at the labels of your personal care products and cosmetics that you already own. Some of your products probably will not have ingredient listings, because the ingredients would have been listed on the original packaging, but work with what you can. If you simply try to say the names of the ingredients out loud, you will probably realize what a chemical soup many cosmetics are. Just realizing what goes into the products that you and your family uses on a daily basis is going to be an eye opener.

First, look for any products that might have the warning label "Warning—The safety of this product has not been determined." That is a good reason to get rid of that product as soon as possible. Next, look up your favorite brands on the Skin Deep Cosmetics Database. Not all of the items that you and your family use might be listed, but it will give you a starting point to find out how hazardous, or how safe, the products might be. If the specific brand is not listed, you can look up ingredients instead. If the products you use contain any of the ingredients from the EWG's list of top chemicals to avoid (*www.ewg.org/skindeep/top-tips-for-safer-products*), start making plans to switch out those products first.

You will probably be okay in using up a specific item and then buying a healthier alternative when it is time to replace that product, rather than throwing everything out all at once. Most of the health hazards come from long-term exposure. But if you have skin sensitivity, allergies, or other health problems that you think might be related to a product, make the switch right now.

Hidden Health Benefits

You might be surprised at the immediate health benefits of using more natural and organic cosmetics, or synthetic cosmetics with a lower health hazard. The chemicals in many of the products that you use on your body could be causing the problems that you buy more products to cover up, such as dandruff, flaky skin, redness, irritation, blemishes, etc. If you switch to a pH-balanced shampoo made of natural ingredients, perhaps your hair will suddenly stop breaking. If you stop using a moisturizer with artificial fragrance, maybe your skin wouldn't be so red and irritated. The possible health benefits are varied, and depend on your special situation and condition. Instead of buying more products to fix the problem, wouldn't it be easier just to fix the cause?

Use Fewer Products

Reduce the number of products that you use, and you will reduce the amount of ingredients that you are exposed to. Regardless of whether you use synthetic or natural cosmetics, there is always a chance that you will have a reaction to something in the long ingredient list. If you find a few great products that multitask, not only will you save time in your daily routine, you will save money, too.

FACT

According to the EWG, every day women use twelve products containing an average of 168 ingredients. Men use about half of that amount, with an average use of six products each day that contain eighty-five ingredients. Children are exposed to sixty-one ingredients each day, on average.

Natural Does Not Mean Risk-Free

Choosing more natural-based cosmetics can have many benefits, but it will have its pitfalls, too. Just like with any cosmetic company, you will find some products that you like and some that you do not. Healthier and more natural-based cosmetic products sometimes have higher price tags because of the expense of the premium ingredients, which can deter you from trying out a brand that you are not familiar with. When trying out a product for the first time, try to purchase it at a store that offers a money-back guarantee on cosmetic items, such as Whole Foods, CVS, and Vitacost (*www.vitacost.com*). Many online retailers with products not found in large retailers will offer money-back guarantees, too. Just be sure to ask about the return policy and understand it completely before purchasing a product that you are testing out for the first time and might want to return.

Plant- or food-based products can still cause a negative reaction. Soy is a common ingredient found in healthier cosmetic items, but many people have allergies to soy. Plant-based oils used in lotions and makeup can cause breakouts if they clog pores. Fragrances from essential oils might cause skin irritation. By reading the labels, you can spot ingredients that might trigger health problems, just like with any other cosmetic item.

Shopping for Cosmetics

By now, you might feel skittish about heading into the personal care aisles of your favorite store. Well, you have every right to be. It should not be so difficult to protect your health when you simply want to buy a bar of soap or a new shade of eye shadow. Though the facts about the cosmetic industry might be a little overwhelming, rest assured that there are a myriad of healthier, safer cosmetic companies out there that make great products.

Pick the Right Companies

Some cosmetic companies are extremely strict about what they put into their products, with only the purest ingredients possible. Others use a combination of healthy ingredients mixed with some synthetics to create their formulations. Many companies refuse to acknowledge the possible links with chemicals and health hazards, though, and use anything that is not illegal. Your challenge is to pick companies with a philosophy about your health and safety that you appreciate, and then start having fun trying out their products. When you understand the rationale behind the ingredients that a company allows to be used in its products, you won't have to worry so much about the ingredients or stress as much about reading labels, though it is always wise to do your research when possible.

ESSENTIAL

There are many companies with a great commitment to producing safer cosmetics. Just a few to check out are Weleda (*www.weleda.com*), Vitacare (*www.vitacareworld.com*), Tom's of Maine (*www.tomsofmaine.com*), Desert Essence (*www.desertessence.com*), Giovanni (*www.giovannicosmetics.com*), Gabriel Cosmetics (*www.gabrielcosmeticsinc.com*), EcoLips (*www.ecolips.com*), and Aubrey Organics (*www.aubrey-organics.com*).

For instance, Burt's Bees (*www.burtsbees.com*), which makes a wide array of personal care products, lets consumers know the exact percentage of natural ingredients that are used in each specific item. Most products are in the upper 90 percent range, with several being 100 percent natural. Not all of the ingredients are of natural origin, but the majority of them are, and that might be fine for you.

If you do not want to settle for anything less than 100 percent natural origin ingredients, a company such as Lily Organics (*www.lilyorganics.com*) is the right fit for you. There are no synthetic ingredients in the company's products, which are crafted by hand each week from ingredients from their own organic farm.

Compact for Safe Cosmetics

The Campaign for Safe Cosmetics created the Compact for Safe Cosmetics, which allowed companies who were interested in producing safer cosmetics with full ingredient disclosure to be recognized. To be a member of the Compact for Safe Cosmetics, companies had to agree with the following six steps set forth by the Campaign for Safe Cosmetics:

1. Comply with the EU Cosmetics Directive.
2. Disclose all ingredients.
3. Publish and regularly update product information in EWG's Skin Deep database.
4. Comply with ingredient prohibitions and restrictions under the Compact for Safe Cosmetics and substitute ingredients of concern with safer alternatives.
5. Substantiate the safety of all products and ingredients with publicly available data.
6. Participate in the Campaign for Safe Cosmetics.

More than 1,500 companies signed the Compact for Safe Cosmetics until the program closed in mid-2011 due to an overwhelming amount of data that had to be processed with each new company. You can use the "List of All Compact for Safe Cosmetics Signers" (*www.safecosmetics.org/display .php?modin=50*) to find companies that have demonstrated a desire to create safer cosmetics.

Every Little Bit Counts

Even if you do not completely switch over to 100 percent organic and natural cosmetics, every change that you make will reduce your exposure to potentially unhealthy ingredients on a daily basis. Every synthetic ingredient you avoid lessens your exposure to chemicals. You might not be able to find a healthier mascara or hair spray that suits your needs, but if you switch as many other products as possible, you can still feel beautiful while doing as much as you can to stay healthy, too.

CHECKLIST FOR HEALTHY COSMETICS

❏ Realize that there is little to no regulation for the cosmetics industry. The concern with products that you use on your skin and body is that no independent party is checking to make sure that they are safe. This is a huge problem, since you use so many items on your body each and every day.

❏ Avoid ingredients that have a high health hazard, according to the EWG Skin Deep Cosmetics Database. Avoiding potentially unhealthy ingredients can reduce your risk to health problems.

❏ Carefully read the labels and marketing claims of all products that you buy. Find out which ingredients are used, and do not be afraid to question claims that do not seem right.

❏ Try to switch to products with safer, more natural ingredients. The more products that you use without harmful chemicals, the less you have to worry about.

❏ Use fewer products to reduce your chemical exposure. Streamlining your products can help you to reduce your chemical exposures, even if you do not buy all natural products.

❏ Find companies with safe ingredient policies that you admire. It's no fun having to read labels all of the time, so find the companies that you feel safe buying products from.

CHAPTER 13

Bedroom

Your bed is the integral part of your bedroom. The mattress itself, as well as the bedding and pillows on top, all work together to create a relaxing place to sleep and unwind after a long day. Since you spend so many hours on your bed over the course of your lifetime, shouldn't it be as healthy as possible? By choosing the right materials, you can create a safe haven that wraps you in luxury every time you lie down at night.

Mattress Risks

You probably spend more time on your mattress than any piece of furniture in your house. Your body recharges and restores itself for the next day's activities while you lie on it. It is likely the largest item in your bedroom and takes up the most amount of space. So shouldn't your mattress get a little extra thought, beyond the color of sheets that you want to put on it, if you want it to treat you nicely?

Fire Retardants

The use of chemical fire retardants is a major concern for many people who want to avoid exposure to questionable chemicals. One class of chemical fire retardants, polybrominated diphenylethers (PBDEs), were banned from use in polyurethane foam products in the United States in 2005. PBDEs have been linked with reproductive system damage, as well as cognitive difficulties and behavioral changes. Though PBDEs are not used in mattresses today, if you have an older mattress that was manufactured before 2005, they could still be in your mattress.

PBDEs are just one type of chemical fire retardant, though. When one is banned, there are others that are used. There are many types of chemical fire retardants in use today on products that you buy, including mattresses and bedding items that have never been adequately tested for human health safety and toxicity.

Why are fire retardants used on mattresses? As of July 2007, mattress sets must meet new federal standards to ensure that the mattress will not burn quickly if it is exposed to an open flame. Preventing mattress fires is not a new concept, though; the CPSC's Standard for the Flammability of Mattresses and Mattress Pads had been in place since 1973. The standards are in place to help prevent fires from lit cigarettes, lighters, and matches that are dropped on a mattress, as well as candles used near a mattress. Though these standards are designed to improve fire resistance and help to slow the spread of flames, they do not make mattresses fireproof.

Though most manufacturers use chemical fire retardants, they are not necessary to meet federal safety standards. The CPSC's "Sleep Safer" publication (*www.cpsc.gov/cpscpub/pubs/560.pdf*) states that "CPSC does not require mattress manufacturers to use fire-retardant chemicals" and "There are compliant mattress sets available that do not use fire-retardant chemicals."

Chemical Exposures

Fire retardants are not the only type of chemical that you can be exposed to while sleeping on a mattress. If your mattress is made up of synthetic materials—and most of them are—any chemicals used in those materials can off-gas and linger in your indoor air. Many of the chemicals are petroleum-based. Formaldehyde is just one example of an unhealthy chemical commonly found in conventional mattresses.

Memory-foam mattresses should be of special concern for anyone who is trying to avoid unnecessary chemical exposure. A Duke University study found sixty-one chemicals present in this kind of mattress, which is made of synthetic foam that conforms to your body. Many people who buy a memory-foam mattress for the first time complain about the odor that the mattress emits, especially for the first few weeks. These mattresses might not let a glass of liquid fall over when placed on the bed, but do you really know what you are inhaling all night long? Manufacturers do not tell you what materials and chemicals are used in the construction of the foam, but don't you want to know?

When to Replace Your Mattress

There is no set rule on when to buy a new mattress, but chances are that you will know when you need a new one. If you feel that your bed is lumpy and uncomfortable, or if you feel like the springs are starting to poke through, then it is probably time to start looking for a new mattress.

You do not need to feel problems in the structure of the mattress, though, to justify a new purchase. You might have put two and two together and realize that your allergies flare up every time that you sleep on your bed, or you are concerned about flame retardants and how they might be affecting your child's behavior. You spend a great deal of time lying on your mattress, so if you feel that it is compromising your health, it is time to start searching for a healthier alternative.

If you have had your mattress for ten years, and have slept on average eight hours a night, you would have spent more than 29,200 hours lying on the mattress. That is the same amount of time as spending fourteen years of forty-hour work weeks on the job (not including weekends)!

Choosing a Healthy Mattress

There is no one-size-fits-all method for choosing a healthier mattress. The firmness or softness of the mattress should depend on your specific needs. Your budget can play a major role in what type of mattress you will buy, including where you purchase it from and what materials are used. Whatever your requirements and your lifestyle, though, there are ways to make this major home investment much healthier and safer.

Types of Mattresses

There are many different types of mattresses made from a variety of materials, which can be either natural or synthetic, including:

- **Innerspring mattress.** The most traditional type of mattress, this type has coiled springs surrounded by layers of cushioning.
- **Latex or rubber mattress.** A latex foam core, whether natural or synthetic, is used instead of coil springs. Natural rubber from the rubber tree is often also called latex.
- **Memory-foam mattress.** Using a visco-elastic memory foam, these mattresses are thick and dense and promise pressure relief and less motion.
- **Futon mattress.** Typically used in beds that fold up for easy storage, futon mattresses are fabric stuffed with synthetic or natural batting materials that bend easily.

Preferable Materials

Natural materials that have not been treated with any chemical fire retardant, fungicide, or other synthetic treatment are the healthiest options for your mattress. You might not be familiar with some of the materials, but they can act in the same ways that the synthetic materials can.

Wool is often used in chemical-free mattresses because it is naturally fire-retardant. Manufacturers who strive to create chemical-free bedding often use wool to meet the federal safety standards for flammability. Wool has many other naturally inherent qualities, too: it is antibacterial, antifungal, and antimicrobial, and it easily wicks away moisture.

FACT

Wool bedding can absorb up to 30 percent of its weight in moisture throughout the night, which will then evaporate during the course of the next day. Synthetic materials only absorb up to 2 percent of their weight in moisture, which often does not evaporate as easily.

Organic cotton is grown without the use of chemical pesticides, so you do not have to worry about pesticide exposure. Cotton is considered the most toxic crop in the world, with cotton growers using 25 percent of all pesticides in the United States.

Natural rubber, also called latex, is not like the synthetic rubber or latex. Milk from the rubber tree is processed into the springy material that you are familiar with. Natural rubber repels mold and mildew and is antifungal, dust mite–resistant, and antibacterial. Natural rubber, unlike cotton, is not highly flammable. Rubber mattresses absorb more motion than innerspring mattresses and conform to your body.

Where to Buy

Mattresses made of all natural materials without chemical fire retardants can be hard to find in common mattress-selling stores in most parts of the country. You likely cannot just walk into your local department or furniture store and try one out. But there are certain areas of the country, such as California, that have more stores offering chemical-free and "green" home goods for customers to try. If you live near a manufacturer of these chemical-free mattresses, there is often a showroom available for consumers to look at the products. You could also contact a manufacturer directly and ask whether there are any places in your area where you could try out one of their beds, such as a bed-and-breakfast or a hotel chain that has purchased mattresses from the company for their guests' use.

You will probably have the most luck finding chemical-free and organic mattresses by shopping online. A number of different manufacturers make a variety of mattresses using natural materials. Lifekind (*www.lifekind.com*) features natural rubber, organic innerspring, and rubber and innerspring combos. Vivetique (*www.vivetique.com*) offers natural latex and innerspring mattresses. Rawganique (*www.rawganique.com*) sells organic innerspring, natural rubber, and organic cotton-wool futon mattresses. CozyPure (*www .cozypure.com*) specializes in natural latex mattresses, including one version with innersprings, while Savvy Rest (*www.savvyrest.com*) features only natural latex mattresses.

QUESTION

How can I buy a mattress without testing it out first?
Mattress manufacturers know that customers are wary of purchasing a mattress without lying on it first. That is why many of them offer return and exchange policies. Look at individual companies to see what their policies are, but many offer free samples and customized shopping assistance to help you pick the right mattress.

Budget-Minded Options

You might be taken aback by the prices of these chemical-free mattresses compared to the least expensive models available at your nearest department store. That is because natural materials are expensive to raise and harvest, while synthetic chemicals mass produced in a lab are cheap.

There are ways to get a healthier night's sleep without breaking the bank, though. If your heart is set on buying a chemical-free mattress, investigate the companies that sell the mattress that you are looking for. Get on their e-mail lists or join their social media pages. Manufacturers often have sales or special offers, such as free shipping, that can bring down the cost. Pay attention for coupon codes or clearance events that can also reduce the expense of a natural mattress.

Perhaps there is no way that your budget can allow for a chemical-free mattress. Do not worry. Investigate the options of traditional mattresses available to you. Some mattresses might have excess chemical finishes, such as antimicrobial sprays, that you do not want. Ask if you can order the mattress without them.

Regardless of what type of mattress that you prefer, much of the off-gassing is going to occur in the first few months, especially if the mattress is coming brand-new from the manufacturer and has been sealed up in a plastic bag. To reduce your exposure to off-gassing chemicals, find a mattress that you like and ask to buy the floor model. It might sound crazy, but you are going to put sheets and possibly a mattress pad or cover on the mattress anyway, and the chemicals would have escaped during the time in the showroom. Buying a floor model might save you some money, too.

ESSENTIAL

Let the chemicals escape from your traditional mattress even more quickly by placing the mattress outside for a few days, especially if you can get it in direct sun. The heat of the sun's rays will heat up the materials, causing chemicals to off-gas faster and release from the mattress before you bring it inside.

Some companies make mattresses with fewer chemical additives than others. The Swedish-born IKEA chain of stores (*www.ikea.com*) has traditionally had less chemical-intensive mattresses for sale to cater to the desires of European consumers, yet is also one of the least expensive choices for mattresses, too. Other well-known brands also have greener options. Serta has an HGTV Green Home by Serta collection (*www.serta.com/hgtv-green-home-mattress-collection-beds-by-serta.html*) that features organic cotton and linen covers and soy-infused foams.

Pillows

Although you are in close proximity every night to the materials within your mattress, just think about how much closer you are to your pillow. Especially if you are a side or stomach sleeper, then your nose and mouth are just inches away from the pillow, inhaling the air that surrounds your bedding throughout the night.

Pillow Allergies

The typical pillows at a big-box store are made from synthetic materials, especially petroleum-based chemicals. Often produced from polyester, synthetic latex, or polyurethane foam, the pillows are cheap, but you are laying your head on a fluffy cocoon of fibers made from chemicals.

There are many pillows available that are labeled hypoallergenic or specifically for allergy sufferers. It is common to have allergies to your pillows, but the solution is not necessarily to switch out one synthetic pillow for another. Many people are allergic to the dust mites that can be breeding in their pillows, which especially feed off of the moisture that gets trapped in synthetic materials. Dust mite encasements can help prevent dust mite allergies in any type of material, but it is even better to get a pillow made from a material that naturally repels dust mites. Even if dust mite allergies are not your problem, it might be chemicals causing the allergies, so switching to another synthetic pillow labeled "hypoallergenic" might not help.

Feather and down pillows can be problems for allergy sufferers, too. Allergies to down are common, but often there is another cause. Because mildew is the real problem for so many people, manufacturers often try to douse the feathers or down inside a pillow with chemical fungicides and mold repellents.

Types of Materials

While chemical-free mattresses are only made from a limited number of materials, chemical-free pillows have a few more options:

- **Wool.** The lanolin in wool naturally repels dust mites, which is great for allergy sufferers. Wool is also naturally resistant to mold, mildew, and bacteria. Wool will compress down by about one-third of the original size.
- **Cotton.** Organic cotton is made without pesticides, but will flatten down considerably over time. If you like soft and fluffy pillows, this choice is not for you.

- **Latex.** Whether small, shredded pellets or a single block of latex foam, latex is naturally resistant to mold, mildew, and dust mites and can offer great support while sleeping.
- **Kapok.** Similar to a down pillow, kapok is the silky fiber from seed-pods of the kapok tree. Unlike down pillows, though, kapok offers more support and firmness.
- **Buckwheat.** Made of tiny buckwheat hulls, these fiber-free pillows are often chiropractor-recommended, since the filling material will move around and naturally cradle your head.
- **Hemp.** Similar to cotton or wool, hemp pillows are made of a natural fiber that will pack down over time to be the slimmest, firmest pillows.

Easy to Buy

Unlike chemical-free mattresses, which can be difficult to find and expensive to purchase, pillows made from all natural materials are much more affordable and readily available at stores where you might already shop.

Chemical-free pillows can start around forty to fifty dollars and are available at the same stores that sell chemical-free mattresses, such as Lifekind (*www.lifekind.com*), CozyPure (*www.cozypure.com*), Savvy Rest (*www .savvyrest.com*), Rawganique (*www.rawganique.com*), and Vivetique (*www .vivetique.com*). They can also be found at some big-name stores, too, such as Amazon.com (*www.amazon.com*) and Bed Bath & Beyond (*www .bedbathandbeyond.com*).

Bedding

Just like mattresses and pillows, the fibers in your bedding, including sheets, pillowcases, blankets, comforters, and duvets, can be a source of chemical exposure unless you are careful about what you choose. Surprisingly stylish options made from all-natural materials are easy to find and becoming more and more affordable.

What to Avoid

If you have a favorite sheet set that you have had for years, you probably do not think there is anything wrong with it—and you may be right. After many washings, a majority of the chemical residues that might have lurked on your bedding are long gone. If you have sheets, blankets, throws, and comforters that you have had for a while and take the proper precautions to keep dust mites at bay, then there is no need to switch to anything else.

When it is time to purchase new bedding materials, though, there are some things that you want to avoid. Sheet sets with "wrinkle-free" or "worry-free" finishes are likely coated with a material that contains formaldehyde. If you do not want to lie on the chemical used to embalm frogs in high-school biology labs, then stay away from these finishes. Same goes with "antimicrobial" or "antibacterial" finishes, which are usually chemical-based. While most of the finish may wash out over time, you can never totally erase it from the bedding's fibers.

Polyester is made from synthetic materials, and cotton, though natural, would have been heavily doused with pesticides while it was growing unless it is organic. The dyes that are used to color fabrics often contain heavy metals, too, although you probably would not know it just by reading the bedding label or even contacting the manufacturer.

Preferable Materials

What kind of material makes a great choice for your sheets without all of the worry? Organic cotton is popular, as is bamboo, which gets softer and softer the more that you use it, creating a luxurious sleeping experience. Linen, which comes from flax plants, is also another choice that gets softer the longer that you have it. Cotton and wool are the best choices for blankets, comforters, and duvets.

Purchasing Healthy Bedding

While it is easier to find chemical-free pillows than chemical-free mattresses, it is ridiculously easy to find chemical-free bedding. Organic sheet sets can be found for sale at many major retailers, such as Target (*www.target.com*) and Pottery Barn (*www.potterybarn.com*). Of course there are plenty of small, niche companies that specialize in organic bedding of all kinds, from sheets to duvets, that have unique and stylish options, such as Magnolia Organics (*www.magnoliaorganics.com*), Gaiam (*www.gaiam.com*), Anna Sova Home (*www.annasova.com*),

Holy Lamb Organics (*www.holylamborganics.com*), and Coyuchi (*www .coyuchi.com*).

Adding Comfort and Protection to Your Bed

If you have a mattress that you like and do not want to get rid of it, there are ways to make it even more healthy and comfortable without great expense. Mattresses and pillows can be modified with chemical-free accessories to create a sleeping environment that fits you perfectly.

Allergen Coverings

Dust mites can thrive in bedding because they live on dead human skin, which sheds onto bedding during the night, and moisture, which tends to get trapped in a bed. While there are many ways to prevent dust mites and their allergenic droppings, you can prevent the creatures from even getting into your mattress or pillow in the first place with a dust mite–proof encasement.

Often called a barrier cloth, these encasements are made of a fabric woven so tightly that dust mites cannot penetrate it. The encasements are similar to a pillowcase and can be slipped over a mattress or pillow and then zipped up, effectively barring the access of any critters. The best barrier covers are made from cotton or wool barrier cloth. Magnolia Organics (*www.magnolia organics.com*) and Rawganique (*www.rawganique.com*) sell encasements.

ALERT

Many allergen encasements are made of polyester, which is made from petroleum and is not good at wicking away moisture, which dust mites thrive on. Barrier covers made from synthetic materials often tend to make noise when touched, such as when you change positions in the middle of the night.

Mattress Cushions and Coverings

Perhaps you want to add another layer of cushiony softness to your existing mattress. Or maybe you need protection from moisture and spills.

Whatever you choose to put on top of your mattress should be as chemical-free as possible, just as your mattress and bedding should be. Many companies make mattress pads out of cotton or wool. Instead of using a pad containing plastics to protect your mattress from moisture, wool moisture-protector pads, with naturally water-repellent properties, can work just as well. Even pillow-top mattress toppers can be made of natural latex, organic cotton, and wool, just like the chemical-free mattresses. The same companies that sell chemical-free mattresses and sheet sets often sell mattress toppers and protectors made out of the same materials.

CHECKLIST FOR A HEALTHY BEDROOM

❏ Choose natural materials such as wool, latex, cotton, and kapok for mattresses, pillows, and bedding. The best way to create a less toxic bedroom is to choose bedding made only from natural materials. Since you spend so much time in bed, it only makes sense that you want the items to be as chemical-free as possible.

❏ Replace your mattress if it is uncomfortable or if you think that it is contributing to health problems. You might not need to replace your mattress right now with a more natural alternative unless you are experiencing problems.

❏ When purchasing a new bed, consider buying the floor model to prevent exposure to off-gassing chemicals. Save money by letting toxic chemicals off-gas in the showroom, and you can bring home the aired-out mattress, which often costs less.

❏ Allergen covers will protect your pillows and mattress from allergy-causing dust mites. Dust mites can cause a lot of allergies, but if you cover your bedding, they cannot survive or thrive.

CHAPTER 14

Babies and Children

When you bring a new child into the world, you want to protect them from everything. The good news is that you can protect them from many of the toxic exposures that are common in daily life. Because of many parents' concerns over the health and safety of items for their children, there is a wealth of chemical-free and nontoxic products available for all aspects of your child's life.

Why Children Have Different Needs

Children are not just mini-adults. From the moment that they come into this world, babies are at risk from a variety of things that adults do not need to fear. Their tiny bodies do not process chemicals the same way that an adult's does, yet little study has been done on the effect of chemicals on a child's development. Most chemical exposure limits for items used in the home are determined by adult reactions, not a child's, which makes it even more important to shield them from the toxic elements of this world.

Rapid Breathing

Babies breathe much faster than adults. Newborns typically breathe forty times per minute, while adults breathe about half that amount or less. More breaths mean more air inhaled into their tiny lungs—and more exposure to any chemicals the air contains.

Developing Systems

Children are more vulnerable to chemicals because their organs and immune systems are not yet fully developed. Without the full strength of their detoxifying organs, such as the liver and kidneys, as well as a reduced response by their immune system, infants and children cannot adequately protect their bodies from harm.

Pound for pound, children's exposure levels to toxins are higher than adults because the concentration of chemical exposure in children is stronger. Children have a higher percentage of body fat than adults while they are developing, and since chemicals are often stored in a human's fatty tissues, that means that a child can have a greater percentage of toxic chemicals in their body compared to an adult's.

Everything Goes in the Mouth

If you have ever watched a baby long enough, you soon realize that everything they touch goes into their mouth. Everything. From toys and toes to cell phones and paper, if children can get their hands on something, chances are it will end up in their mouths. The desire to suck and chew on objects that they find can be especially hazardous to children, because many of the items were never designed to be ingested, so health studies have never been done on the residues or ingredients of those products.

Even if a child does not put a foreign object in their mouth, they are likely to put their hands in their mouth, which can harbor unhealthy particles and debris. Babies and children crawl on the ground, where they are in close proximity to pollutants and chemicals that accumulate on the floor from shoes and naturally occurring dust. Even the great outdoors can be a source of chemical exposure if a child touches a lawn or plants that have been sprayed with toxic materials.

Inherited Chemicals

Children are not born into the world with a clean bill of health, though. The Environmental Working Group has found an average of 200 chemicals and pollutants in umbilical cord blood, including fire retardants, Teflon chemicals, pesticides, stain-resistant coatings, and car emissions. Many birth defects are now believed to be caused by exposure of a genetically susceptible embryo or fetus to environmental toxins.

Cribs and Bedding

When you bring your baby home from the hospital, chances are that she will spend more time in her crib than in your arms. As your child gets older, she will spend a lot more time in bed than you do, with longer sleep times at night, as well as naps throughout the day. Whatever materials are used in your child's mattress and bedding will have a deeper and longer exposure to their body compared to the materials used in yours.

Mattresses

Mattresses can contain a slew of chemicals, from toxins used in the foam to synthetic fire retardants sprayed on the fibers. These ingredients can be harmful to adults, so they can be especially problematic to children, who sleep in very close proximity to the mattress materials for ten to fourteen hours a day. Of even greater concern is the fact that young children are exposed to so many brand-new mattresses during the span of a few short years. Chemicals in mattresses off-gas much faster during the first few months of use. A new crib mattress is often purchased right before a baby comes, which means the chemicals used in the materials are still fresh and coming out at a high rate. Then, when it is time to move to a big kid's bed, a child-size mattress must be bought, usually brand-new again. If you did not buy a twin-size mattress when making the transition from a crib to a bed, then another mattress must be bought yet again when your child grows even more.

When buying an organic mattress, do not be misled by marketing claims. You want to find a mattress made entirely of organic cotton, wool, or natural rubber, preferably with no chemical fire retardants added. While cotton should be labeled as organic, wool or natural rubber will likely not be labeled as organic but will still be safe. Products that simply have an organic cotton cover are not as healthy as those made with all-natural ingredients.

Chemical-free mattresses are widely available for cribs. While it can be hard to find nontoxic mattresses in queen and king sizes for adults, parents' strong demand for nontoxic items for their children mean that organic and all-natural child-size mattresses are a lot easier to find. The prices are not too terribly bad, either. Organic crib mattresses often sell for about $100–$300, which is a lot less than the cost of an adult-sized bed.

ESSENTIAL

Chain stores such as Babies "R" Us (*www.toysrus.com*) and Target (*www.target.com*) offer organic crib mattresses, making it easy to add to your baby registry as a gift that someone can buy you. Specialty retailers offer a great selection of organic baby mattresses, too, such as Lifekind (*www.lifekind.com*), Pure-Rest (*www.purerest.com*), and Dax Stores (*www.daxstores.com*).

Cribs

Just as important as a chemical-free mattress is a chemical-free crib. The structure that you set the mattress in should contain no harmful chemicals that will off-gas directly into your baby's sleeping area. Pressed woods are notorious for containing formaldehyde-containing adhesives that release not only formaldehyde, but also many other toxic vapors.

When choosing a crib, determine what materials it is made from. If the crib is produced from pressed woods, engineered woods, or MDF, be wary about the synthetic chemicals that can be released from the item, especially if you are buying it brand-new, because the chemicals will off-gas even faster in a new product. Solid wood cribs, especially unfinished woods without any synthetic stains or sealants, are ideal.

ALERT

Be careful when using or buying secondhand cribs. Older cribs can be especially unsafe because they do not meet strict updated safety requirements. More than 11 million cribs have been recalled since 2007, and drop-side cribs are now banned because of safety concerns. However, many of these cribs are still available through resell avenues, even though they are unsafe.

If you truly want to avoid the toxic chemicals in a crib, you can use an old-fashioned Moses basket as your child's first bed. These narrow, handled baskets are often made from natural palm leaves and have a simple mattress made of organic materials inside. Heart of Vermont (*www.heartofvermont .com*) creates an organic version of these beds. Moses beds are much easier to keep clean, because they can be disassembled quite rapidly, and are highly portable during your baby's first months, allowing your baby to sleep wherever you carry her.

Bedding

If you buy an organic mattress, it only makes sense to use organic bedding on top of it. Your baby's sensitive skin will be in direct contact with the bedding for hours every day. Cotton sheets are grown with massive amounts of chemical pesticides; you can avoid them by choosing organic cotton sheets. Polyester is made with petroleum by-products and is not very good at wicking away moisture, creating a hot, damp sleeping environment for your little one.

As with mattresses, there are plenty of organic choices for baby and toddler bedding nowadays. From bumper pads and swaddle blankets to sheets and dust ruffles, the options are varied and available in major retail stores such as Pottery Barn Kids (*www.potterybarnkids.com*) and Walmart (*www .walmart.com*), as well as specialty retailers such as Magnolia Organics (*www.magnoliaorganics.com*) and Under the Nile (*www.underthenile.com*).

Diapers

Your baby will use approximately 6,000 diapers before becoming toilet-trained. That is a lot of diapers that come in constant, direct contact with your baby's skin. Clearly you must use diapers, but the ones that you choose can make a big difference in your child's health.

Disposable Diapers

Parents around the world rejoiced when the first disposable diapers were introduced. No more having to wash dirty diapers, and plenty of convenience when traveling or away from home. Compared to the previous cloth diapers, though, disposable diapers do come at a price.

Disposable diapers are expensive as well as horrible for the environment, since it takes 200–500 years for a disposable diaper to decompose—or so scientists think—because diapers have not been around long enough for anyone to know for sure. The diaper that your child is wearing right now will still be in a landfill when his great-grandchild ten times over is born.

FACT

There are disposable diapers that are a little kinder on the environment and potentially on your child's health because of the materials that are used. Disposable diapers such as Tushies (*www.tushies.com*) and Tender Care Diapers (*www.tendercarediapers.com*) use less toxic ingredients such as a chlorine-free wood pulp fluff inside the diaper, and many are fragrance- and latex-free.

Because of their plastic-based components, disposable diapers can cause health problems for your child. Synthetic plastics can contain a vast array of chemicals that will be in contact with your child's skin every hour of every day of every month of every year before they are potty-trained.

Disposable diapers often also contain dyes, fragrances, and chlorine that can irritate your child's skin.

A study published in 2000 in the *Archives of Disease in Childhood* found that scrotal temperature was significantly higher in boys wearing disposable, plastic-lined diapers than in boys wearing cloth diapers. Since hot temperatures can adversely affect the creation of sperm, the researchers recommended further research on whether male infertility might be exacerbated by the types of diapers worn in childhood.

Cloth Diapers

There is a new generation of cloth diapers that are easier to use and care for. No longer are there just squares of cotton that must be secured with a safety pin, although those products still exist. Now there are fitted cloth diapers with hook-and-loop or snap closures, as well as diapers made from eco-friendly materials such as hemp, bamboo, or organic cotton. These diapers come in a wide array of colors and prints. Often, the diapers have a removable or flushable liner, such as gDiapers (*www.gdiapers.com*), and Kushies (*www.kushiesonline.com*), to make cleaning easier and a little less gross for the parents.

ESSENTIAL

While choosing your diaper choice, keep in mind your choice of diaper wipes, too. Diaper wipes commonly include propylene glycol (a binder also found in antifreeze), parabens (commonly used as preservatives), and synthetic fragrances. Choose wipes such as Seventh Generation (*www.seventhgeneration.com*), which are chlorine-free, whitened without chlorine bleach, unscented, and alcohol-free, but still get the job done.

Cloth diapers are a great alternative to plastic disposables, but quite honestly are not always the best alternative. Children could still have a reaction to the wetness of a cloth diaper or the detergent used on the diapers. After all, in the quest to be chemical-free, a cloth diaper does not work as well if it is washed in harsh detergents by a diaper-cleaning laundry service.

When trying to choose between cloth and disposable diapers, consider using cloth diapers at home and disposables for day care and trips away from home.

Bottles

Your baby's first nutrition often comes from a bottle, whether you use formula exclusively or breastfeed and often have to store milk in a bottle. Baby bottles and sippy cups can be made with plastics that contain potentially toxic chemicals that can leach into the liquids that your baby drinks. With some smart shopping on your part, you do not have to worry about exposing your child to these dangers.

BPA

Bisphenol-A (BPA) is a plastic additive that hardens plastic and makes it transparent. BPA is only found in plastics with a recycling symbol number 7, but not all number 7 plastics contain BPA. Because plastics containing BPA are nearly shatterproof, they were often used in baby bottles and other infant feeding items.

FACT

A baby's BPA exposure does not just come from a bottle. A 2007 study by the Environmental Working Group found BPA in 33 percent of cans of concentrated soy- and milk-based infant formulas. These formulas come in cans lined with plastics and epoxy resins that can contain BPA. Powdered formulas might be a safer alternative in preventing exposure to BPA.

BPA can come out of the plastic and into the liquid stored inside a baby bottle. Since BPA is considered an endocrine disruptor that has also been linked with obesity, diabetes, early onset of puberty, and cancer, that is not a good thing. BPA comes out of plastic at a faster rate when hot liquids are placed inside or when a bottle has been exposed to high temperatures, such as putting the bottle in the dishwasher for proper cleaning. If the bottle is scratched or chipped, BPA can be released even faster.

BPA-Free Plastic Bottles

It is possible to enjoy the convenience of nonbreakable plastic baby bottles without the worry of BPA exposure. Many companies, such as BornFree (*www.newbornfree.com*) and ThinkBaby (*www.thinkbabybottles.com*) make BPA-free plastic bottles. Just walk down the baby products aisle of any store and you are likely to see many varieties with bold marketing labels stating that they are BPA-free. Plastics made from another variety of plastic other than #7 will not contain BPA, either.

Glass Bottles

In the quest to avoid toxins, plastics are always a concern. For truly chemical-free alternatives, glass bottles are an ideal choice. Glass bottles are not necessarily fragile items that can be easily broken, though you do still have to use common sense. Many glass baby bottles come with plastic overlays that help protect the glass and allow baby to grip the bottle, such Evenflo's (*www.evenflo.com*) shatterproof glass bottles. Glass bottles are better for infants; for active toddlers, who often throw things, BPA-free sippy cups are ideal.

Food

How many times have you said to a child that they need to eat right so that they can grow up strong and healthy? Parents say those wise words because they are true. Yet eating right goes beyond just eating more fruits and vegetables. It also means that whatever food your child is eating should also be chemical-free.

Choosing Organic

When it comes to buying food for your baby, perhaps you have seen an increase in the amount of organic items that are now offered for children.

Why are organic foods so popular for children nowadays? It is because an organic designation means that the food contains ingredients that have not been grown with chemical pesticides or fertilizers, an important distinction for parents who are trying to limit their children's toxic exposures.

Organic foods are also free from genetically modified organisms (GMOs). Still relatively new on the scene, GMO foods are genetically engineered to contain their own pesticides to prevent pests or have some other artificial change to the DNA of the crop. These foods are not a product of nature. The effects of GMOs are not well known, because they have only been around for a decade or so. Unfortunately, many of the crops that are part of the American diet are already genetically engineered, such as many soy, canola, and corn crops. The only way to avoid these products is to buy organic or look for labels that claim GMO-free.

Simple Ingredients

Organic foods are not always widely available, and they can be costly. What is a parent to do, then? Read the labels and choose only foods that are made from ingredients that you can pronounce and understand what they are. In his book *In Defense of Food: An Eater's Manifesto*, food activist and author Michael Pollan says, "Don't eat anything your great-grandmother wouldn't recognize as food." This dramatically simple advice recognizes the fact that much of the food available now is full of lab-created chemicals. Great-Grandma would not have recognized cream-filled snack cakes or pink yogurts with candies on top, and chances are they aren't too good for you now.

In keeping with the back-to-basics mantra, try to skip foods with chemical additives and altered ingredients, such as high-fructose corn syrup, trans fats, artificial colorings and flavorings, and artificial preservatives that just are not necessary. There is just no logical reason that children's drinks should be bright blue, that their cereal should be neon pink, or that their snacks should have a shelf life of more than three years.

Make Your Own

To truly know what goes in your child's food, it is best to just make it yourself. Whether you are making pancakes from scratch instead of buying the frozen kind, or pureeing fruits and veggies to create fresh baby food, you can control exactly what your child eats. Not only is there a wealth of cookbooks available to teach you how to make nutritious meals for infants, toddlers, and older kids, but there are also gadgets and kits such as Beaba's Babycook (*www.beabausa.com*) and the Baby Bullet for making baby food quickly and affordably.

Toys

Your child will put everything he sees into his mouth, whether it is supposed to be there or not. While you might be concerned about your child putting items into his mouth that are not toys, the shocking truth is that some of the toys designed for children's playtime can be just as dangerous, as well.

Phthalates

Plastic toys are made of a cocktail of chemicals to make them soft and flexible. PVC (polyvinyl chloride) is widely used, and many PVC products contain plasticizers or phthalates, chemical compounds, which make the plastic more flexible. Phthalates are of great health concern because they have been potentially linked to cancer, hormonal disruption, early puberty, and reproductive defects.

In 2009, the CPSC set a standard for toy manufacturers that no toy could contain any more than 0.1 percent of six types of phthalates, though testing for phthalates in toys did not start until 2010. The decision came ten years after the European Union banned six phthalate plasticizers from children's toys designed for kids younger than three. Even before the new toy standard, though, Walmart and Toys "R" Us declared in 2008 that they would stop selling toys that contain phthalates.

Even though toys that contain the six phthalates should not be available to children anymore, they might still be. Toys that do not adhere to the new safety standards, as well as older toys that were purchased before the new standards took effect, can still contain potentially toxic phthalates.

Stick to the Basics

When purchasing toys for your children, especially ones that are designed to go in their mouth, it is wise to stick to time-tested materials that have been used for generations. Solid wood toys make a surprisingly healthy alternative and, no, you do not need to worry about splinters. Wood toys that are untreated, unfinished, and unpainted are safe to chew on because they have no toxins to leach out and no toxic paint or sealant residues. Companies such as Three Sisters Toys (*www.threesisterstoys.com*), Melissa and Doug (*www.melissaanddoug.com*), and Uncle Goose (*www.unclegoose.com*) are among the modern-day manufacturers who are continuing the tradition of wooden toys.

Toys and dolls made of organic cotton and wool are also safe and are especially great for small children who suck on toys, since they can be laundered in the wash. From cloth balls to stuffed dolls and everything in between, there are a variety of cloth-based toys for children of all age levels.

CHECKLIST FOR CHILDREN'S HEALTH

- ❏ Choose mattresses and bedding made from organic and natural materials. Your child will spend a majority of their day sleeping, with their tiny noses pressed against the bedding. Make sure it is as healthy as possible by choosing chemical-free bedding.
- ❏ A crib should be made of solid wood to prevent off-gassing chemicals. If you buy organic bedding, do not let chemicals coming from pressed wood cribs ruin the healthy environment that you are trying to create.
- ❏ Disposable diapers that use less chemical ingredients are available for convenience. Diapers made with wood pulp or not bleached with chlorine can cause less irritation than traditional disposable diapers.
- ❏ Consider hybrid cloth diapers, which have replaceable inserts. Allow only the natural fibers of cloth to touch your baby's skin, while also getting rid of the ick factor of using cloth diapers, by using hybrids instead.
- ❏ Use BPA-free baby bottles and sippy cups. The hormone-disrupting chemical can leach out of bottles and sippy cups and affect your child's developing health.
- ❏ Feed your children with fresh, natural foods. A growing body needs vitamins and natural ingredients as fuel, not processed or synthetic ingredients.

❑ Make foods from scratch whenever possible. Processed foods will contain more preservatives and other stabilizers than fresh foods.

❑ Avoid plastic toys and choose wood and cloth ones instead. Plastic toys, just like plastic kitchen items, can leach chemicals when sucked or chewed on.

CHAPTER 15

Pets

If you have a dog or a cat or another type of furry companion at home, you know that they are not just animals. They are a part of your family. You want them to live a healthy and long life, too. But pets can experience health problems from items in your home just like humans can. In fact, your four-legged family member might be more vulnerable to toxic products at home than you would have imagined.

Why Pets Are More Vulnerable

Based on your pet's behavior, you might have a hard time thinking that he could ever be affected by a few chemicals in the home. After all, he eats dirt, grooms himself in the most private of places, and might even bring you some nasty treats from outside. Yet with all of pets' unsavory habits, they can still have delicate systems that need care.

Close Exposure

Pets are in closer proximity to problematic items in your home than you might realize. Dust and toxins that accumulate on the floor and in fibers of a rug can be unhealthy to anyone in a home. A pet, however, is much closer to the floor and can inhale more of these substances than a person. The same is true for cleaning products, lawn care products, and more.

Eating Everything

Not only are pets closer to potential toxins, but they also consume more of them. Indoors, pets have a tendency to lick floors to pick up bits of food or water, which means they are also licking up the dust and residues that have been left on the floor from cleaning or from daily foot traffic.

ALERT

Even though medications help to keep you healthy, those medications can be a source of poisoning for your pet. Human medications were again at the top of the ASPCA's "Top 10 Pet Toxins" list for 2010, and can include sources such as ibuprofen and acetaminophen. Always keep medications secured in places where your pet cannot access them.

Pets also eat a lot of stuff outside. From dirt and sticks to plants and puddles of water, pets are not afraid of ingesting what they discover in the great outdoors. If those items have been treated with chemical sprays and other treatments, your pets will directly ingest the toxins.

Common Household Toxins

There are some things in your home that can be harmful to you, but are likely to be even more toxic to your pets. Preventing exposure to household items that might actually be poisons is the first step in creating a healthy home for your pet.

Lawn Care and Pest Products

According to the ASPCA Animal Poison Control Center, about one-fifth of the calls that they receive are about possible poisonings from insecticides. Rodent traps and herbicides also round out the list of the top ten pet toxins. These products can be harmful to children and humans, too, so it is especially important to keep fertilizers, bug killers, and weed killers stored in proper containers out of reach of pets. Do not allow pets to be in the same room or outdoors when you apply a bug killer or other product, and allow the product to dry before your pet has access to the area.

Cleaning Products

You might think that household cleaners smell bad, but your dog or cat might think otherwise and want to eat the product. Regardless of whether you use a nontoxic cleaner or a chemical-laden one, always keep cleaning products stored out of reach of pets in proper containers with the lids securely fastened.

Pets are not just exposed to cleaners in the bottle, though. Pay special attention that your pet does not drink water from a newly cleaned toilet bowl or lap up detergent from an open dishwasher door. Just-mopped floors, as well as newly polished furniture, can also lead to cleaner exposure in your pets.

Antifreeze

Your car needs antifreeze in the cold winter months, but this common product is especially problematic to pets. Because antifreeze often has a sweet taste, pets are more apt to lick it up if they find a spill.

To protect your pet from exposure, be sure to wipe up any drips and spills that might occur in pouring the product into your vehicle. You can also purchase a different type of antifreeze that is more pet-friendly. Antifreeze made from ethylene glycol is considered the most dangerous because it has an appealing smell. A less-hazardous antifreeze is made with propylene glycol, which can still be dangerous but has a bitter taste that might prevent your pet from lapping up the product.

Plants

You would not think that plants could pose a health hazard to pets, since pets spend so much time outdoors where they are surrounded by the natural elements. But quite a few plants can be poisonous to pets that chew on the branches or ingest the leaves.

ALERT

Flower bouquets can be a source of toxins to pets. For instance, lilies can be especially toxic to cats. If you have a vase of flowers for a special occasion, display the bouquet in a place where your pet does not have access to the flowers.

Both indoor and outdoor plants can be toxic to pets. The ASPCA has a list of "Toxic and Non-Toxic Plants" (*www.aspca.org/pet-care/poison-control/plants*) that can be searched by name and picture. You can find plants that are toxic to cats, dogs, or horses, as well as clinical symptoms of exposure to the plant.

Toys

If you have ever watched a dog excitedly run again and again after a tennis ball, you know how much a pet can love playing with toys. Toys are important for mental stimulation and exercise, but choosing the right kind of toys can also be important to reduce your pet's toxic exposures.

Chemical Exposures

Have you looked in a pet toy aisle lately? Were you overwhelmed by the amount of bright colors, squeaky inserts, and molded plastic forms of all shapes and sizes? Pet toys have become very synthetic. All of the plastics that are used to create tiny balls with bells inside and large flexible dog bones and everything in between are mostly made of chemicals. And they all go into your pet's mouth.

Just as with children's toys, soft, flexible plastics contain a chemical compound known as a plasticizer. Usually these plasticizers are made of chemicals called phthalates, which are shown to disrupt the endocrine system. While some phthalates are banned from children's products, especially ones that would go in their mouths when they are young, there is no ban on phthalates in pet toys.

Lead is another problem with pet toys. Though there is great concern about lead in children's products, pet toys do not get the same respect. In tests done by the Washington Toxics Coalition and the Ecology Center, one in four of the 400 pet products tested had lead. Tennis balls for pet use were more likely to contain lead, and nearly half of all tennis balls tested had lead levels, though tennis balls for human sports use did not have lead. Seven percent of the products tested had lead levels higher than what the CPSC allows in children's products.

Eating While Playing

Ever notice how quickly a pet can tear apart a toy? That is why pet stores sell so many toys that are guaranteed not to fall apart or be torn up. Demolishing toys is not just a financial concern; it can be a health concern, too, because as the toys are torn apart, small amounts of the product are ingested by your pet.

Even if your pet has never torn apart her toys, the toys are still always in her mouth. After the licking, pulling, and chewing, whatever ingredients are in your pet's toys are in direct contact with their mouth. If these chemicals can be released from the product, they will be ingested.

Healthy Alternatives

Cats can be entertained by a piece of jute string for hours. Many dogs enjoy simply chomping on a stick. It does not take much to create a toy for a pet. Sometimes the best things are free and easily available.

If you want to buy toys for your pet, look for ones that are as chemical-free and natural as possible. Purrfectplay (*www.purrfectplay.com*), Simply Fido (*www.simplyfido.com*), West Paw Design (*www.westpawdesign.com*), and Chewber (*www.chewber.com*) are some great options.

Sleeping Areas

Your pet probably spends a large portion of his day lying around. Why not create a healthy place for your pet to lay his head? Nontoxic options are easy and inexpensive, but can have a dramatic effect on the quality of your pet's health.

Nontoxic Bedding

Just like a human's bed, pet beds can be made with all kinds of synthetic materials that can off-gas chemicals or be sprayed with toxic fire retardants. Since pets are not as picky as humans about their beds, it is especially easy to find nontoxic alternatives for them.

First, start with the basics. Would your pet be okay with just a sheet or blanket balled up into a pile? Many pets like to dig into a blanket and maneuver it to fit just right. It is especially easy—and cheap—to find a simple blanket made of all cotton or wool or an old comforter that you are not using anymore.

If your pet demands a more plush bed, or if you want one that fits better with your stylish decor, there are still plenty of nontoxic options for your pet's sweet dreams. Avoid buying any bed made from polyurethane or synthetic foam. These manmade materials can off-gas chemicals into your pet's breathing space. Instead, look for beds stuffed with natural ingredients, such as cotton, buckwheat, or wool, that have not been treated with chemicals. Some great options are West Paw Design (*www.westpawdesign* *.com*), PurrfectPlay (*www.purrfectplay.com*), LifeKind (*www.lifekind.com*), and Olive (*www.olivegreendog.com*). You can also easily make a pet bed by sewing two squares of fabric together and stuffing with cotton or wool batting or old towels and comforters.

ALERT

Be wary of any pet bed or other pet product that claims it is "antimicrobial" or "antibacterial." Unless these products are made from natural wool, chances are that they have been sprayed with antibacterial chemicals, such as triclosan, which can possibly be unhealthy for your pet.

Dust Mites

Pets can suffer from dust mite allergies just like their owners do, but their reactions can be dramatically different. People usually suffer from upper respiratory symptoms due to indoor allergies, but pets have a different response, which usually includes excessively itchy skin that can then lead to serious health problems such as infections and hair loss.

To limit your pet's exposure to dust mites, wash pet bedding in hot water at least once a week to kill the health offenders. Vacuum regularly, including upholstered furniture. If your pet lies on your bed, be certain to wash your bedding in hot water once a week, too.

Bathing and Grooming Products

A smelly dog probably is not a healthy dog, but a dog bathed with the wrong cleaners might not be healthy, either. It is important to choose nontoxic products that will not irritate your pet's skin and will not leave toxic residues that can be ingested later.

Sodium Lauryl or Laureth Sulfates

Sodium lauryl sulfate (SLS) and sodium laureth sulfate (SLES) are very common ingredients in soaps and shampoos, both for pets and for humans. Just because they are common, though, does not mean that they cannot cause problems. These detergents, which are used to make a product have suds, are commonly being tied to skin and eye irritation. There are plenty of natural ingredients that can be used in a soap or shampoo other than SLS and SLES to create suds without health effects.

Other Harmful Chemicals

SLS and SLES are far from being the only chemicals in pet-grooming products. Parabens, phthalates, and artificial fragrances also show up in these products, even though they are not necessary. Unfortunately, pets can react to these chemicals in the same ways that humans do, which means endocrine disruption, allergies, and more.

Buying Healthier Products

There are many ways to clean your pet without resorting to synthetic ingredients. There are plenty of items on the market that promise organic and natural ingredients. Be sure to read the labels and determine if what you are getting is truly as all natural as you want, since marketing claims can be confusing and tricky, just like with any other home product that you might buy. Among some wonderful options are Aubrey Organics (*www.aubrey-organics.com*), Vermont Soap (*www.vermontsoap.com*), and Spa Diggity Dog (*www.spadiggitydog.com*).

Homemade Pet Shampoo

You can also make your own shampoo for your pet, too, if you really want to control what is in it. Though there are many variations on home-made shampoos, here is one recipe to try:

- 1 cup dish soap
- 1 cup apple cider vinegar
- ⅓ cup glycerin
- 1 quart water

Mix all of the ingredients and use just like a shampoo. Keep in mind that there are no preservatives in this recipe, though, so you will not want to keep it lying around for a very long time.

Flea and Tick Control

No one likes to deal with fleas or ticks. Not you. Not your pet. Fleas and ticks can bring with them some serious health problems that should not be taken lightly, but traditional, chemical solutions to flea and tick problems can have their own health risks, too. There are ways that both you and your pet can be chemical-free, as well as tick- and flea-free.

Legal Pet Poisons

It takes a pesticide to kill fleas and ticks. After all, these creatures are living pests. So any time that you use a flea or tick control product on your pets, you are dousing them with pesticides. The challenge is in finding natural remedies that can work like pesticides without the chemical exposure.

A study by the Natural Resources Defense Council found that many flea and tick control products leave behind toxic residues, sometimes for weeks. Chemicals that could cause cancer or damage the neurological system were found in some collars at levels nearly 1,000 times higher than the EPA allows in products for children.

FACT

Toxic chemicals used on pets are not just a health hazard to the animal. Children play with pets and then put their hands in their mouths, ingesting any residue that was found in a pet's fur. Adults are at risk, too, with exposure to petting an animal and then unknowingly touching their eyes or mouth.

Many pesticides are banned in use of pet products, but there are still toxic chemicals, such as propoxur, that are allowed to be used. The state of California has banned the use of propoxur, which it classifies as a known human carcinogen, though the EPA and other states have not followed suit. Other chemicals that the Natural Resource Defense Council suggests to avoid in pet products are amitraz, fenoxycarb, permethrin, and tetrachlorvinphos (TCVP).

Some chemicals have already been removed from pet care products because of health concerns. They include chlorpyrifos, dichlorvos, phosmet, naled, diazinon, and malathion. As of 2006, these chemicals should no longer be in your pet's products. But if you have really old products lying around, or if you have access to pet care products that still contain these chemicals, keep in mind that the chemicals are now considered unsafe for both pets and humans.

Natural Solutions

Using chemical-free options to keep fleas and ticks at bay might require a little more work on your part, but it will greatly reduce you and your pet's exposure to toxic chemicals. Among the most effective ways to reduce the number of fleas and ticks is to check your pet's fur frequently. A fine-tooth comb drawn through your pet's fur will make fleas and ticks stand out, where they can then be caught. Put the fleas in a small bowl of soapy water, and they will immediately die.

Washing and bathing your pet is another great way to naturally kill fleas. Fleas will die in soapy water, whether you pick them off and put them in the soapy water or the soapy water comes to them in a bath. Do not use flea and tick shampoos with chemical ingredients, though. Fleas will die with just plain old dish soap, so do not expose your pet to chemicals when they are not needed. Choose a gentle soap that will not be harsh on your pet's skin or leave chemical residues behind.

Just like washing your pet's bedding in hot water will kill allergy-causing dust mites, laundering will also kill eggs and larvae, too, plus any adult fleas that are found in the bedding. Vacuuming is also another highly effective solution, just as when dealing with dust mites, to round up the bugs and their eggs and get rid of them. If you have a large problem, consider using a steam cleaner, using just the hot water steam to kill the fleas without any chemical additives.

Finding Less Toxic Options

Trying to find a less toxic product to kill fleas and ticks can be a little difficult, but it will be worth it for the health of your entire family. The Natural Resource Defense Council has a "GreenPaws Flea and Tick Products

Directory" (*www.simplesteps.org/greenpaws-products*), which lists pet products by name so that you can find out what chemicals are used in the ingredients and the possible toxic effects. You can also print out a wallet card (*www.greenpaws.org/_docs/GP_pocketguide.pdf*) that lists which chemicals to avoid.

Sometimes natural remedies might use essential oils to repel pests. Whether these products work for you will depend on your pet's tolerance of the oil. Among the most gentle oils are:

- Cedarwood
- Peppermint
- Rosemary
- Thyme
- Lemongrass

Neem oil, made from the seeds of the neem tree, is a potent oil that can effectively control pests on plants, humans, and animals. Neem oil can often be found in pet products to use for flea and tick control, but just like with any ingredient, it must be used carefully and watch for signs of intolerance.

Take Care of the Lawn

Besides treating your pet and the indoors, you need to take care of the outdoors, where fleas and ticks breed. Keep your yard tidy, without too much overgrown brush or unkempt plants. Fleas and ticks like to hide in shady, moist conditions, so dry, sunny locations without much cover are less likely to be breeding grounds.

Treat your yard with flea and tick controls, too, in order to kill the pests. As with products designed for use on your pet, look for natural ingredients. Neem oil is often used in outdoor applications.

Cat Litters

Of special concern to cat owners is cat litter. Most indoor cats need a litter box, but there can be health problems associated with this product. Of course, you want to find a product that can deal with the odor problem effectively, too. As always, the best solution is to find the least toxic ingredients that work for you.

Clay Ingredients

Traditional cat litters are made with bentonite clay. This clay, while natural, is nonbiodegradable and requires strip mining to acquire. When you pour this cat litter into a litter box, you have probably noticed clouds of dust. That dust is made of silica, which is a known carcinogen.

You obviously do not want to inhale a known carcinogen, and your pets should not inhale it, either. Your cats probably do not want to eat it, but that is just what happens. Cat litter can get stuck on their paws, then they groom themselves, and before you know it they have ingested the product. Because clay cat litter will not break down or biodegrade, the cat litter can build up in your cat's digestive system and potentially cause serious health problems, not just from chemical exposure but also due to obstruction of the digestive system.

Better Alternatives

While clay cat litter is the most widely known type, there are alternatives. Feline Pine (*www.felinepine.com*) is made of biodegradable pine shavings that are reclaimed from lumber production. The pine oils that could otherwise cause sensitivity are removed, leaving behind a much healthier cat litter. Arm & Hammer (*www.armandhammer.com*) makes a cat litter out of unused corn cobs, along with baking soda. These are just a few examples of the natural ingredients that can be used to create cat litter. Other ingredients often used are recycled newspaper, oat hulls, wheat, and alfalfa.

CHECKLIST FOR A HEALTHY PET

❑ Control your pet's access to common poisons, such as medications, cleaners, and lawn and garden products. Pet poisonings are most often caused by items commonly found around the house. Be careful about what your pet can get into, and choose nontoxic alternatives to reduce the risk.

❏ Be very careful with antifreeze leaks or spills during the winter, and purchase a more pet-friendly version. Antifreeze is necessary in the winter, but the sweet taste of antifreeze that is not contained properly is often lethal for pets.

❏ Avoid using toxic plants to pets indoors or in outside landscaping. Even though they are natural, some plants can be harmful to pets if ingested.

❏ Choose pet toys made from natural materials. Many dogs end up eating small bits of their toys, so make sure that they will not ingest harmful plastics.

❏ Wash pet bedding frequently in hot water. Pets can have dust mite allergies, too, so kill the bugs with hot water.

❏ Choose pet beds made from natural materials and not synthetic foam. Synthetic foam can off-gas chemicals into the air surrounding your pet's bed.

❏ Choose chemical-free grooming products. Pets can be affected by chemicals in grooming products just like humans can, but all-natural alternatives work just as well.

❏ Try to prevent fleas and ticks in natural ways before resorting to sprays. The least toxic way to control fleas and ticks is to prevent them from entering your home and reproducing.

❏ Choose the least-toxic flea- and tick-control option that will work for you. Sometimes you will need a chemical-based remedy to kill fleas and ticks, but start with the least toxic method available.

❏ Avoid cat litters made with clay. Clay-based cat litters can cause digestion problems, as well as releasing harmful dust into the air.

CHAPTER 16

Pest Control

Pesticides can be bad, but that doesn't mean you have to spend your next picnic with mosquitoes biting your arms, ants nipping at your toes, and wasps buzzing around your head. Exposure to insects has health risks, too, but there is a broad middle ground between doing nothing to control pests and dousing your yard with toxic chemicals that carry a slew of health warnings.

Products Designed to Kill

There is a spray or powder to kill just about anything that manages to live in your yard or come into your house. Notice the word "kill." These products are designed to put an end to living creatures, so doesn't it make sense that they might have a few health risks for you, too?

Problematic Chemicals

There are many chemicals that can be used in a pesticide for bug-killing power. With so many different chemicals, it is hard to research how these chemicals can interact with each other, to say nothing of the long-term health consequences after years of exposure. The pieces are starting to fall together, though, and the results do not look good, either for public health or the health of the environment.

QUESTION

How can I find out more about the chemicals in pesticides?
There are several search engines that allow you to look up a certain chemical by name and learn more about toxicity levels, health risks, etc. The Pesticide Action Network (*www.pesticideinfo.org*), Beyond Pesticides (*www.beyondpesticides.org*), and the National Pesticide Information Center (*http://npic.orst.edu/index.html*) have extensive information on the health and safety hazards of chemicals.

The EPA oversees pesticides based on the Federal Insecticide, Fungicide, and Rodenticide Act (*www.epa.gov/oecaagct/lfra.html*). But as with cosmetics, the EPA does not actually test the products for safety; it relies on the testing performed by the companies themselves. Toxicity tests of ingredients often rely on results about exposure to a single chemical in high doses. These tests do not take into account long-term doses of low levels or how the chemical might react with another chemical.

Inactive Ingredients

You might think that you could just look at the ingredients label of a pesticide and find the chemicals that kill the pests, and then try to choose among your options for the least toxic ingredients. That is good thinking, but laws do not give you that option.

FACT

The EPA started a "Enable the Label Discussion Forum" (*http://blog .epa.gov/enablethelabel/*) in 2010 for anyone who is interested in learning about and discussing the ideas of pesticide labeling. The blog breaks down the EPA's Pesticides Label Review Manual into easy discussion topics each month and encourages the public to leave comments and responses.

Pesticides also contain inert ingredients, which do not have to be listed on the bottle. These are not the actual killing chemicals, but work in conjunction with them by acting as a bait or propellant or by allowing the chemical to adhere better. In many cases, the inert ingredients can make up more than 99 percent of the pesticide. The EPA even says about the products, "Called 'inerts' by law, the name does not mean nontoxic." Acetone, butane, kerosene, and propane are just a few of the inert ingredients that can be included in your pesticide without your knowledge.

You might not be able to find out the inert ingredients in a pesticide, but that does not mean that there are not health risks. The toxicity of many inerts used is unknown, but several have been studied and have been linked to health risks, such as cancer and reproductive damage.

Overuse by Homeowners

While there is often great debate over the use of pesticides on food that we eat, the reality is that homeowners often create pesticide problems at home, too, in the quest for the perfect lawn. The EPA has found that seventy-eight million homes use pesticides each year, with more than ninety million pounds of pesticides applied to homes and yards. The numbers are staggering enough, but when put into context with the agricultural industry, landscaping sales of pesticides are nearly four times greater, and homeowners use up to four times as many applications of pesticides per acre as the agricultural industry.

Methods of Exposure

Pesticide manufacturers have long stood behind the claim that pesticides are only used to kill bugs, and that people are not exposed to health risks because they are not directly exposed to the chemicals in the pesticides. The products that you apply to your grass, though, have a sneaky way of finding their way into other places where they shouldn't be.

Aerosol Sprays

Many indoor insecticides come in an aerosol can or spray bottle, allowing you to spray from a safe distance and still hit your target. The problem with spray cans of bug killer, though, is that the insecticides quickly become airborne and contaminate the air inside your home. In fact, up to 98 percent of spray insecticides end up somewhere other than the intended target. An EPA study found that the air inside a home contained at least five pesticides at concentrations more than ten times greater than that of outdoor air.

ALERT

Baits can be a healthier alternative than sprays or liquids, because they do not as readily become a part of the indoor air. But even solid pesticides can eventually become a part of your indoor air. If you have children or pets that could get into the baits and ingest them, the health risks are still high.

Toxic Surfaces

Toxic residues from bug sprays can linger on indoor surfaces, such as floors and kitchen countertops, for a very long time. The places where insects roam and pesticides are applied are the exact same surfaces where you walk and cook food.

The makers of chemical-based insecticides have long claimed that the products are safe if used correctly. Have you ever stopped and looked at the back of an insecticide bottle lately, though? Many products that might be used in a kitchen warn of first removing all dishes, cookware, food, and even shelf liners from the area that you are spraying before applying the pesticide, then letting it dry while you leave the room, then washing the surfaces down before reusing. If an insect is running across the counter while you are preparing dinner, are you really going to ask it to stop while you can prepare the area so that you can spray a bug killer, then clean the area before resuming dinner preparations?

Direct Exposure Outdoors

Outdoor pesticides can have a direct source of exposure if you touch an area treated with pesticides with your bare hands, feet, or skin, or if any item treated with pesticides, such as leaves, grass, or soil, is ingested. This method of exposure is especially problematic with children, who put their hands in their mouth frequently, or pets, who groom their fur and paws and can then ingest the chemicals.

Some of the most potent doses of pesticide exposure come at the time when you are mixing or applying the pesticide. Large amounts of the chemical product can give off dangerous and toxic fumes that can be inhaled, while skin exposure to the product directly can cause poisoning and burns. Without using proper safety precautions, mixing and applying pesticides can be risky.

How Outdoor Pesticides Get Indoors

Most pesticides are designed to be used outdoors and stay outdoors, but this does not happen. If your yard is sprayed with a pesticide, there will be some residue left behind, even after it dries. Then you walk across your lawn and patio and get that residue on your shoes. Then you walk inside your house. Now there are pesticides inside, where they can become embedded in carpeting fibers or other areas of your home. Pesticides can also come into your home if the windows are open and you, or your neighbors, are applying pesticides outdoors.

A study published in *Environmental Science and Technology* found that after a lawn pesticide application, chemicals drifted into a home and were tracked in, creating levels of the chemicals that were ten times higher than before the pesticide application.

Human Health Problems

Though pesticides are never supposed to affect people, more and more studies suggest that pesticides do indeed affect human health. You do not need to be a farmer, a pesticide professional, or even the person in your home who applies the pesticides to be affected.

Long-Term Risks

Beyond Pesticides' "Health Effects of 30 Commonly Used Lawn Pesticides" fact sheet (*www.beyondpesticides.org/lawn/factsheets/30health.pdf*) states that out of thirty common pesticides used on the lawn, nineteen can possibly cause cancer, twenty-one can have reproduction effects, eleven have the potential to alter your hormonal system, and thirteen are linked with birth defects. Pesticide exposure is thought to possibly contribute to many health problems such as:

- Alzheimer's disease
- Asthma
- Birth defects
- Cancer
- Diabetes
- Learning disabilities
- Parkinson's disease
- Reproductive problems

Poisoning Risks

The warning labels on pesticide bottles that say "DANGER," "WARNING," or "CAUTION" are there because of the short-term health dangers that can be caused by pesticides, such as skin and eye irritation and deadly poisoning. You must take proper precautions when using pesticides to prevent these immediate health risks.

If you think that you or any member of your family might have swallowed, inhaled, or have had your skin exposed to pesticides, it is important to call the American Association of Poison Control Centers at (800) 222-1222, or your local poison control center, for help in diagnosing and treating the problem. The National Pesticide Information Center at (800) 858-7378 can also answer nonemergency questions on the phone and offers a handy card (*http://npic.orst.edu/PesticideEmergencyCard.pdf*) to print out with emergency numbers that you should know.

ALERT

The EPA's "Emergency Information" (*www.epa.gov/pesticides/health/emergency.htm*) warns that "Eye membranes absorb pesticides faster than any other external part of the body; eye damage can occur in a few minutes with some types of pesticides." The EPA suggests to wash an eye exposed to pesticides with clean running water for at least fifteen minutes and to avoid using eye drops in the water.

Do not induce vomiting in a person who has swallowed a poison unless emergency personnel have told you to do so, because some products will cause more damage if they are vomited back up. Pesticide exposures to the skin should be washed quickly and thoroughly with soap and water, unless you are advised otherwise. If you have inhaled pesticides, get into fresh air immediately.

Children at Risk

Among those that are most vulnerable to pesticides are children, because of their increased exposure while playing in the yard and the tendency to ingest more products than adults do. The National Academy of Sciences has estimated that half of a person's lifetime exposure to pesticides comes before the age of six. Home and garden pesticides are thought to increase the risk of childhood leukemia by as much as seven times, while the chemicals are also linked to behavioral disorders and developmental delays.

Fix the Causes First

If you have a bug problem, chances are your first reaction is to grab a pesticide. But pesticides should always be the last resort. Many of the bug problems that are common in a home and outdoors can be eliminated without any bug-killers at all by simply blocking a pest's entry points or destroying their homes.

Seal Off the House

The most effective way to deal with an insect problem inside is to first seal off the entry areas that the pests are using. You will not have a pest problem indoors if the pests can't get in. Gaping cracks and unsealed doors are like throwing open the door for the insect world to enter. You will probably greatly reduce your pest problems without the use of any pesticides by simply sealing cracks and entryways in places such as windows, doorjambs, floorboards, and molding, and any other nook and cranny where you might notice a place where insects and rodents could enter. Use caulk or weather stripping to seal all of the gaps and openings around windows and doors to prevent a tight seal that insects can't easily get through. Mesh netting on windows and screen doors can prevent pests from flying right into your home, but only if there are no rips or tears. When looking for insect entry points into your home, look both indoors and outdoors, especially all around the base of your home's foundation. Also be sure to remove clutter, whether indoors or against the house. If pests do not have a place to hide, they can't.

Remove Food Sources

So much of what draws in bugs from the outside can be found in the kitchen. Sugar, starches, trash, and leftover food particles are all what tempt bugs to pack up their belongings outdoors and move inside to greener pastures. Rethink the kitchen and the rest of your home from a bug's point of view. Take a critical look at everything, from floor to ceiling, and consider whether it might be a food source for a pesky insect that you have been dealing with. Dog food left in a bowl overnight, a bowl of cough drops, fruit that is going bad, crumbs on the couch, or even a child's craft project made of dough or macaroni might be drawing in bugs. Remove potential food sources to quickly and easily take care of your pest problem. Keep trash covered in trash bins outside.

Wipe down with an all purpose cleaner the surfaces in your kitchen that might unknowingly harbor food residues, including the inside of kitchen cabinets and drawers, all around the stove, and under the refrigerator and dining room table. For open packages of food products, purchase air-tight containers to store the food and pet food.

ESSENTIAL

Store dry goods, such as rice, flour, sugar, and pasta, inside the refrigerator. These starches often draw bugs. Insects do not like the cold temperatures of the refrigerator and won't find their way inside. The products will cook just the same as when they are stored in the cabinet, plus they will have a longer shelf life.

Problem Plants

Bugs are attracted to plants for a variety of reasons. If you have a major bug infestation outside, you might want to reconsider the items used in your landscaping. Certain plants are just designed to attract certain insects. For instance, if bees are your problem, do not plant nectar-rich plants in your yard. If you are trying to get rid of caterpillars, do not plant species, such as milkweed, that caterpillars live on and thrive off of before turning into butterflies. Trying to kill off insects that you are unknowingly attracting is just a waste of time and energy.

Sometimes insect problems occur because of poor soil. Unhealthy plants can create an ideal environment for insects to grow. Remove diseased and rotting plants from your yard. Cultivate healthy soil through the addition of compost and other organic material to keep problematic pests at bay.

Rethink the plants that you have in your yard. If they are too high-maintenance and require too many pesticide applications to stay healthy and bug-free, perhaps they should be replaced with more native plants or easier-to-care for varieties that do not attract as many bugs.

Cut Off the Water Supply

Pests need water, and even a small leak can provide a source for their survival indoors. Fix leaky plumbing under the kitchen sink, in the bathroom or anywhere else to reduce pest problems. Seal off cracks around water-based sites in your home, such as the toilet and tub, where pests might be able to find residual amounts of water.

Some pests need water to live in. Mosquitoes breed where there are standing pools of water in which their larvae grow. Get rid of the water and you will keep new mosquitoes from forming. It does not take much water for mosquito larvae to grow, so take a look around your yard and dump any standing water, including water in pails and children's toys, pet bowls, rain gauges, fountains that are not running, birdbaths, the tops of garbage containers, etc. Be vigilant about dumping standing water every few days, especially after heavy rains.

Alternative Ways to Kill Pests

Even after you seal off and remove the sources of food and shelter for pests, you might still have a problem. There are ways to prevent bug problems and kill bugs using only items that you can already find in your home.

Dish Soap

Plain old dish soap is a highly effective way to kill ants. Use a few drops of dishwashing soap in a small spray bottle of water and just spray on the ants. It should work almost immediately, so if the ants do not die in a few seconds, add a little more soap to the mixture and try again. Since soap is something that you use to clean your house with anyway, there is no toxic residue left behind. This works well for ants on patios, walkways, and other surfaces, but the soap could harm vegetation.

Food Safe Ingredients

Items that you have at home for cooking can actually be a great pest deterrent, too. For an ant problem, you can try using red chili powder, paprika, or dried peppermint around the areas where ants are entering your home. Peppermint essential oil will also work, too, and adds a pleasant aroma to the home. The insects do not like these ingredients and they will prevent pests from entering into your home in the first place.

For cockroaches and silverfish, there are several ways to make a trap to catch these creatures using food. One idea is to rub some shortening inside the neck of a jar and set upright with a banana inside for bait. Place a popsicle stick or tongue depressor inside from the lid to the banana and then dispose of the insects after they have been caught. Another method is to soak a rag in beer and place in a shallow dish overnight. Dispose of the insects in the morning.

FACT

There are many food-based and plant-derived ingredients that are actually considered "active" ingredients by the EPA in many pesticides, such as mint oil, rosemary oil, thyme oil, corn gluten meal, soybean oil, lemongrass oil, garlic, cloves, cinnamon, geranium oil, cedar oil, and white pepper.

People Power

Often, it might just be easier to kill the bugs as you see them instead of investing in a long-term combative approach. Indoors, kill pests as they occur. Invest in an old-fashioned fly swatter to kill bugs; elbow grease is always nontoxic.

Outdoors, for small insect infestations, pick the bugs off of the plants and dispose of them, instead of relying on a product to kill them. For some bugs, all you need to do is knock them off of the plant, which can be done with a strong spray of water from a spray bottle or the hose. Of course, these methods mean that you need to spend a little more time in your garden looking at your plants, but isn't that the whole point of having a garden?

Less Toxic Pesticides

There are many effective, less-toxic alternatives out there to kill bugs without jeopardizing your own health. Keep in mind, though, that "natural" pesticides can still be toxic if not used properly. Unless you are using preventive techniques, or simple kitchen ingredients such as food or dish soap, pesticides, even plant-based varieties, are still designed to kill and will have an element of toxicity. Choose the least toxic, safest alternative that works for you, be careful with its usage, and be vigilant about keeping pets and children away.

ALERT

Buying Pesticides

There are companies, such as EcoSMART (*www.ecosmart.com*) and Orange Guard (*www.orangeguard.com*) that make pesticide products from naturally derived or plant-based ingredients. With other products, though, marketing claims might lead you to believe that they are natural when they are not. Labels on all brands of pesticides can be very confusing, so always investigate the ingredients to be sure that you know what you are getting.

Natural Remedies

Neem oil, processed from the seeds of the Indian neem tree, is an all-natural bug repellent that works wonderfully and is often used in the garden, as well as in pet products, to help control pests.

Boric acid, which is derived from natural elements in the earth, is a highly effective insect killer, especially with cockroaches. Boric acid is all-natural, but it can still cause health problems, especially with children and pets, but it really does work and is less toxic than many other products on the market. Use it sparingly and cautiously.

ALERT

Diatomaceous earth is another product from nature that works well at killing bugs. It is made of soft, sedimentary rock that is actually composed of the fossils of freshwater organisms. The rock is crushed into small particles that will cut and kill pests that crawl over it, such as snails and slugs. Diatomaceous earth does still have health hazards, though, especially among children and pets, and it is wise to wear a mask when applying it so that you do not inhale the sharp little pieces.

Choosing the Right Pesticide

Not every bug or rodent can be treated with the same type of product. Each insect will be killed in a certain way, so there is no point in exposing yourself to pesticides that will not even work on the offender. Regardless of what type of pesticide that you choose, always make sure that it is designed to kill the bug that you want to kill. Beyond Pesticides offers a list (*www.beyondpesticides.org/alternatives/factsheets/index.htm*) of common insects and the many ways to kill them, listing nontoxic and less-toxic alternatives.

Hiring a Professional

Sometimes a job is too big for you to do on your own. Sometimes chemical pesticides might be necessary, no matter what other steps that you have taken. When it is time to call in someone else to handle the problem, look for a company that can take care of pests in a manner that you think is safe.

Integrated Pest Management

Professionals who utilize the concept of Integrated Pest Management (IPM) use a variety of methods and commonsense practices. An IPM professional might first look around your house for entry points or nests that you were not aware of or could not see. An IPM professional should then offer you several options, some chemical-based, some not. Beyond Pesticides has a Safety Source for Pest Management search engine (*www.beyondpesticides.org/infoservices/pcos/findapco.htm*) or you can do an Internet search for your area with the keywords "Integrated Pest Management" or "IPM."

No Need to Kill Everything

Many service providers want to sell you monthly or quarterly pest control packages so that they can keep coming back and making money, but keep things in perspective. Once you step outside your door, you are in nature, whether it is an urban city sprawl or five acres of wooded farmland. To try to kill off all bugs that exist in nature is both highly impractical and highly illogical. And it can be just plain toxic. If you do not have a demonstrated pest problem, then do not try to kill bugs that are not bothering you.

Investigate Your Existing Services

Perhaps you think that no pesticides are being applied to your lawn, but it's possible your lawn care company has been spraying your yard with pesticides without telling you. Maybe someone who comes into your home to clean is applying pesticides to keep bugs at bay. The rug cleaning professionals might have a pesticide in their cleaning solution that you are not aware of. Pesticide exposure can take place at your home without you knowing it, so it is vitally important to always ask questions of any service provider that you use and determine what is in the products being applied in your home.

CHECKLIST FOR HEALTHY PEST CONTROL

❑ Eliminate or reduce your use of chemical-based pesticides. Pesticides can get into your home and into your body in more ways than you might realize. Prevent exposure in the first place by using products made without harsh chemicals.

❑ Choose less-toxic pesticides made from plant-based ingredients. You can control pests with products made from certain natural ingredients that are less toxic than many chemicals.

❑ Do not allow children or pets to come into contact with materials treated with pesticides. Kids and animals are more susceptible to health problems from chemical exposure than adults.

❑ Block entry for pests by caulking and sealing cracks around your home. If a pest cannot enter your home, it won't.

❑ Remove pests' food sources to control an insect problem. Eliminating their food means that pests will move on.

❏ Remove plants that can be attracting pests. You may be unknowingly encouraging pests with certain items in your landscape.
❏ Hire an Integrated Pest Management professional for major problems. IPM professionals work to look at the whole picture of how to get rid of pests for good.
❏ Do not treat for pests if there is not a problem. Do not waste your time or money spraying to prevent possible future pests.
❏ Always use appropriate safety measures with pesticides, even less-toxic pesticides. Even natural ingredients can be harmful, so always take proper precautions.

CHAPTER 17

Lawn and Garden

Whether you walk barefoot across your grass, your kids eat tomatoes straight off the vine, or your pets love to dig holes in the yard, all members of your family have a more intimate exposure to the plants in your lawn and garden than you might think. Keeping your lawn and garden healthy and happy does not have to be complicated, and it certainly does not require chemicals. In order to enjoy the great outdoors with less worry, start with what you spray and spread across your landscape.

Weed Killers

No matter how great your gardening efforts are, there is a very good chance that you will still need to deal with weeds. Even with all of the preventive measures that you can use, those little suckers still find a way to survive anyway. Since weeds must be managed frequently and consistently, it is important to find a nontoxic solution to reduce your repeated exposure to chemical killers.

What Are Herbicides?

Weed killers or herbicides are designed to kill plants, whether they are tiny weeds that grow in cracks or large patches of poison ivy, when applied to vegetation or soil. Some herbicides are selective, which means that they kill only certain types of plants and let others live. Other herbicides are non-selective, which means that they will kill anything that they touch.

FACT

More than $14 billion is spent on herbicides worldwide each year, with the United States accounting for more than one third of the spending, according to the EPA. In 2007, two billion pounds of herbicide were used on land around the world, with 531 million pounds of herbicide used in the United States.

There seems to be a chemical weed solution for every surface that you can touch in your garden. Herbicides are often added to mulches or soils to prevent weeds, in addition to sprays and granules that you can spread on your lawn or plant beds. Any product that you use outside that says "prevents weeds," "pre-emergent herbicide," "kills weeds," or "destroys all vegetation," will contain an herbicide, even if you are not buying the product to act as an herbicide. The only exceptions are products that block sunlight, such as barrier cloths. That is why your exposure to the ingredients in weed killers can become so high, and why you want to use healthier alternatives instead.

Is Killing Weeds Harming You?

Though herbicides are designed to kill plants and not animals, they often have the same health risks and methods of exposure as pesticides. Keep in mind that the many varied chemicals that are used in herbicides—and there are a lot of them—are designed to kill living things, too.

The U.S. National Library of Medicine warns that herbicides can often contain glyphosate, a poisonous ingredient that can cause breathing difficulty, dizziness, drowsiness, vomiting, and anxiety, among other symptoms. Glyphosate has long been under attack for possibly causing health problems ever since the company Monsanto introduced it in 1974. New studies have linked the chemical with spontaneous abortions, infertility, and malformations in animals. The chemical has been found in the urine of farmers and their children, but the EPA is still re-evaluating its stance on the chemical.

The use of glyphosate is widespread. The chemical is used in the top twenty-five bestselling herbicides and can be found in 750 U.S. products. In 2007, farmers used eight times the amount of glyphosate that they had used in 1992, more than 88,000 tons of the stuff, according to the U.S. Geological Survey Office (USGS). The USGS has found the herbicide in public waterways and air samples.

FACT

Using chemicals to kill weeds can cause herbicide resistance. More than 130 types of weeds show herbicide resistance in the United States, more than in any other country around the world. It is estimated that nearly eleven million acres of farms are affected by glyphosate-resistant weeds.

The weed-killing chemicals such as glyphosate are not the only problems, though. A French study at the University of Caen found that the inert ingredients in the product Roundup, which typically had not been thought to cause harm, can actually kill human cells, especially cells in embryos, the placenta, and the umbilical cord.

Natural Solutions

Weeds in your garden do not need to be killed with chemicals. They can be killed using natural remedies with food-safe ingredients that will not expose you, your family, and your pets to harsh ingredients. Often these natural solutions will cost much less. The most effective solution, which happens to be free, is to simply pull weeds by hand. If you do not have a major infestation of weeds, it could be easier just to pull the offenders that you see before they have a chance to set seed and reproduce.

Preventing weed seeds from seeing sunlight helps reduce their growth, too. Thick layers of mulch, about two to three inches thick, naturally inhibit weed growth, insulate the plants, retain moisture, and organically enrich the soil. For even more weed control, place three or four sheets of newspaper on the soil before adding mulch on top. The newspaper naturally blocks weed growth and will decompose over the course of the growing season.

Products that you would expect to see in the kitchen can also squelch weeds. White vinegar is an excellent weed killer. Spray undiluted vinegar on weeds when the sun is out and they will die within hours. The hotter and sunnier the location, the better. Vinegar is not a selective herbicide, though, meaning that it will kill whatever it touches. Kitchen vinegar has 5 percent acidity, but you can buy industrial-strength white vinegar with a 10 or 20 percent acidity that will kill weeds and vegetation very effectively, though you must take proper safety precautions with the high acidity solution. Corn gluten meal also acts as a natural pre-emergent herbicide and prevents weed seeds from germinating. Both corn gluten meal and industrial-strength vinegar can be found in specialty lawn and garden stores, farm-supply stores, or at Marshall Grain Co. (*www.marshallgrain.com*).

Every year, there are more and more options for naturally derived, eco-friendly lawn and garden products available at major garden centers and home improvement stores. Look for companies such as EcoSMART (*www.ecosmart.com*) that state "naturally derived" or "plant-based" ingredients. Don't be misled by the marketing claims of products that can be very harmful to your health. Always wear a mask when spraying or applying herbicides, even the natural kinds, since inhalation of these ingredients could cause irritation.

Fertilizers

The spiel for pesticides and herbicides applies to synthetic fertilizers, too. Harsh chemicals can have some serious health effects in addition to causing soil, water, and air pollution. It's not necessary to use a chemical sledgehammer when a gentler natural remedy will do.

Surprising Ingredients

Did you know that what gets flushed down your toilet can end up as fertilizer for your fruits and vegetables? According to the EPA, "Biosolids are the treated residuals from wastewater treatment" and "the U.S. Department of Agriculture, the Food and Drug Administration, and EPA . . . endorsed the use of biosolids on land for producing fruits and vegetables."

Human waste is not the only surprising thing being spread on your veggies. Industrial waste is also used, too, some of which is considered hazardous. According to the EPA, "Industrial waste materials are often used in fertilizers as a source of zinc and other micronutrient metals" and "hazardous wastes are used as ingredients in only a small portion of waste-derived fertilizers." So hazardous waste, which by definition is too toxic for a landfill, can be repurposed into a fertilizer used for crops? Perhaps that is why fertilizers often contain levels of many different forms of toxic heavy metals.

Addicted Plants

Ironically, using a synthetic fertilizer on your lawn and garden just creates less healthy plants. Plants thrive on nutrients found in the soil from naturally decomposing elements. When you fertilize a plant with synthetic chemicals, those chemicals strip the soil of naturally occurring microorganisms that help keep the soil healthy. Synthetic chemicals also alter the pH level of the soil, which further stresses the plant. Now the plant is devoid of nutrients and struggling to survive in conditions that it is not adapted to. You will have to keep fertilizing the plant just to keep it alive because it can no longer fend for itself, creating more work for you and an increased dependency on chemicals.

Natural Alternatives at Your Garden Center

There are plenty of options for naturally derived fertilizers that are healthier for your plants and work to enrich and improve the soil, too. Bags of compost or composted manure can be blended with your existing soil to add nutrients and increase beneficial microorganisms. Many prepackaged varieties of fertilizers, whether sprays, granules, or mixes, are available in garden and home improvement stores and through web retailers such as Monrovia Organics (*www.monrovia.com*), Bradfield Organics (*www.bradfieldorganics.com*) and TerraCycle (*www.terracycle.net*). Seaweed, fish meal, and compost teas are also naturally derived nutrients.

Turning Trash Into Treasure

Many of the items that you throw away every day can be used in the garden to naturally help nourish your plants. One of the best ways to turn your trash into treasures for your plants is to compost. There are all kinds of varieties available nowadays, from outside composting heaps you build yourself to self-contained systems you can store in an apartment. You can even buy worm composters that produce nutrient-rich compost "tea." Whichever kind suits your needs, composting is a great way to turn your daily trash, such as paper, food products, and garden waste, into a rich soil amendment that is packed with nutrients and will naturally fertilize your plants while reducing landfill waste at the same time.

ESSENTIAL

Starbucks' Grounds for Your Garden program offers anyone free five-pound bags of used coffee grounds. The used coffee grounds, which would otherwise be sent to a landfill, are packaged daily and usually placed in a bin where customers can grab a bag or two before heading out the door.

If you do not compost, you can still use common items from around the home to feed your plants. If you are a coffee drinker, you can save the used coffee grounds and add them to your soil as a natural fertilizer. Coffee grounds are slightly acidic, so use them for acid-loving plants, such as blueberries, hibiscus, holly, etc. Used tea bags and tea leaves can also be added to the soil.

Cut-up pieces of a banana peel are a great soil amendment for roses. Just place the peel under the soil and let it decompose. What about all of that water that is dumped down the drain after straining pasta or cooked vegetables? That cooking water is actually nutrient-rich and is great for fertilizing plants. Allow the water to cool to room temperature before applying to the base of plants.

Lawn Equipment

Unless you hire someone to do your lawn work or it is taken care of by your homeowners association, chances are you have a lawn mower, trimmer, or leaf blower lurking somewhere in your garage. There are several different types of lawn equipment available for purchase, and as you can imagine, some varieties are much better than others.

Belching Exhaust Fumes

You probably would not stand behind a running car for too long because you would not want to be exposed to the noxious fumes coming out of the tailpipe. So this interesting tidbit might really upset your lawn care routine— a traditional gas-powered lawn mower emits more air pollution than the average new car.

A gas-powered lawn mower can emit as many VOCs in one hour as a car does after driving forty-five miles. Now think about it: Would you walk behind a car and breathe in those fumes for forty-five miles? Obviously not, because you have heard how unhealthy it is. You, your spouse, or your kids might be exposed to the same amount of airborne pollutants, though, after just one hour of weekly lawn mowing, and if you have a big yard that takes more than an hour to mow, your exposure will be higher.

If you are using gas-powered lawn equipment of any type, including mowers, leaf blowers, and edgers, this can be a serious problem. That's especially true for anyone with respiratory problems, as VOCs have been linked with allergies and asthma, as well as eye, nose, and throat irritation, fatigue, and headaches.

The obvious way to quickly eliminate these toxic exposures is to stop using gas-powered lawn equipment. There are other alternatives out there, and while gas-powered lawn equipment is typically used for heavy-duty jobs that need bursts of power, you might want to seriously consider whether your patch of grass needs that amount of power and the health risks that come with it. If you must use gas-powered equipment, do not allow children to be outdoors with you when they are in use. Keep your windows closed when anyone is using gas-powered lawn equipment in your yard or in your neighbor's yard. Cancel a yard service that uses gas-powered lawn equipment and look for a nontoxic alternative instead.

Electric Equipment

You do not have to have smelly, dirty fumes coming out of a piece of lawn equipment to keep your lawn looking nice. Electric lawn equipment has come a long way in the past few years and is readily available in all home improvement stores. Unless you live on a very large tract of land, an electric mower can easily keep the grass cut, while electric leaf blowers, weed eaters, and trimmers can keep the yard neat and tidy.

Electric lawn equipment comes in two different styles—corded or rechargeable cordless batteries. Your choice depends on your situation. If you have electric outlets easily available outside, a corded option means that you do not have to wait for a battery to charge before using the equipment. Rechargeable cordless equipment is great if you do not have access to electric outlets, or do not want to be encumbered with a cord following you around.

An electric lawn mower takes about five dollars of electricity to use each year. That is quite a bargain compared to the amount of gas and oil that it takes to fuel gas-powered equipment. Electric lawn equipment does not require engine tuneups or oil changes, and a push-button start means there's no need to yank on a cord to get it going. With no oil or gas to use, you will not have to worry about spills in the driveway or garage. It also might be easier to listen to your favorite music on your headphones while operating electric lawn equipment because the noise is about half of that of gas-powered items.

Good Old-Fashioned Elbow Grease

There used to be a time when electric lawn equipment was only a dream and gas-powered mowers were a newfangled invention. How did people take care of their lawns then? Using equipment that has clearly stood the test of time.

Though the leaf blower is now the method of choice in clearing paths and walkways, you don't need fancy equipment to get rid of dirt and debris. A broom works just as easily.

What about leaves in the yard during the autumn and winter? A leaf blower will quickly get rid of the problem by pushing the leaves somewhere else for you to take care of them. A rake effectively removes leaves and debris, too, and helps you get you some exercise in the process.

Old-fashioned push lawn mowers are making a big comeback these days, too, and are ideal if you have a small patch of grass that does not take too long to take care of. Many big-name home improvement stores carry push mowers, or you can order online at sites such as Clean Air Gardening (*www.cleanairgardening.com/reelmowers.html*), Amish Lawn Mower (*www .amishlawnmower.com*) and Reel Mowers Etc. (*www.reelmowersetc.com*). If nothing else, they are a great conversation starter among your neighbors.

Professional Lawn Care

Perhaps you do not have the time or physical ability to take care of your own lawn, or maybe you are stuck with a lawn care regimen that is mandated by where you live. Either way, you still have options to keep your lawn from being a toxic dumping ground.

Hiring a Service

While not as readily noticeable on the streets as the lawn equipment companies that pull gas-powered lawn equipment in big trailers behind large trucks, there are businesses that specialize in using eco-friendly and nontoxic lawn care options. You might have to hunt a little bit to find them, but they are there.

ALERT

When searching for "nontoxic" lawn care, you must be very careful to fully understand what types of materials are used. Many companies claim that they use "nontoxic" products because they have not been proven to cause health problems, but the treatments are still full of synthetic chemicals. You need to know what is important to you, and don't fall for marketing claims.

Your first place to look for these services is on the Internet. Most of the time, companies that use electric equipment, manual lawn equipment, or organic lawn treatments are small and do not have the funds for extensive advertising. You can start by first seeing if you have a Clean Air Lawn Care (*www.cleanairlawncare.com*) franchise near you. These companies use solar- and wind-powered electric lawn equipment and organic lawn treatments. On the Beyond Pesticides website (*www.beyondpesticides.org/safetysource/index.htm*), you can also search for companies that use less toxic weed-killing options.

You can also search for other companies by doing an Internet search with the name of your city or area and the keywords "electric lawn care," "nontoxic lawn care," "eco-friendly lawn care," or "chemical-free lawn." You might find a company's website or mentions of suitable companies on discussion boards or gardening blogs.

If you cannot easily find a lawn-care service on the Internet, start asking around to find healthier lawn-care services. A great resource is a nursery or garden center with a commitment to sustainable gardening and organic plants. Ask if they have a list of businesses or people that use electric or manual lawn equipment or green lawn-care products. Perhaps there is a community bulletin board with business cards posted, or brochures by the registers. If you do not have luck asking at garden centers, you can also try calling your local cooperative extension office (*www.csrees.usda.gov/Extension*) for ideas.

When the Choice Is Not Yours

If you live in an apartment complex or have a homeowners association, you might find that it is more difficult to have the types of lawn care that you would like. When another company or a committee is choosing what happens to your lawn, opinions can differ on what is necessary and what is healthier. You can influence those decisions, though, with proper education and community support.

If you are not happy with the type of lawn service that is being provided for you, contact the appropriate people and discuss your concerns. Bring literature that showcases the health risks of chemical-laden lawn treatments to children and pets. Look for examples of how other apartment buildings, condo complexes, or housing developments have made the switch to greener lawn care options and how it has been a positive experience. Have a suggestion for different businesses or specific products to use. If you know what these companies and services cost, that information can help strengthen your case, especially if they are less expensive than what is already being used.

If you are the only one fighting for the change, see if you can get your fellow neighbors to join the cause. Discuss the health concerns from toxic lawn care, and ask if they, their children, or their pets have any health problems that could be linked to the lawn treatment. Your neighbors are paying fees to live there, too, and the more people who are upset, the more likely that a change will be made.

Eco-Friendly Landscaping

The more eco-friendly that your landscaping is, the less hassle it will be. By using plants and gardening techniques that work in cooperation with your soil type and weather, instead of constantly fighting it, you will find that you have to use less artificial sprays to encourage plants to grow. You will also need less weed killer if you have a healthy lawn and garden that naturally chokes out weeds, and you won't even need to worry about hiring a lawn service or taking care of your lawn if there is no lawn, or little lawn, to take care of.

Native Plants

To reduce your chores and time in the garden, use more native plants. Native plants are defined as plants that naturally occur in a particular region or habitat without human intervention. That sometimes includes plants that might not have originally been found naturally in your area, but are highly adaptive to your climate. Because these plants can exist without human contact, they are strong and resilient and will not need much care from you.

As you can imagine, the native plants of Oregon are going to vary dramatically from the native plants of Georgia because of differences in climate, elevation, and soil. The good news is that it is very easy to find what types of plants are native to your area. Each state has a native plant society that can detail what native plants grow in certain regions of your state. PlantNative (*www.plantnative.org*) has a search engine in which you can find the organizations and nurseries that can teach you more about native plants suitable for where you live.

ESSENTIAL

The Lady Bird Johnson Wildflower Center at the University of Texas at Austin has a comprehensive online search engine (*www.wildflower.org/ plants*) that can comb through a list of 7,188 native plants to find the right ones for your state or region and specific gardening needs, such as full sun or moist shade, as well as bloom times and average height.

Native plants also help wildlife in your area by providing familiar food sources and shelter for the butterflies, birds, bees, and other wildlife that are common in your area. Do not be surprised if you start seeing more butterflies flitting around your garden after you install native plants into your landscape.

Xeriscaping

Xeriscaping (zer-i-skaping) is a word that means landscaping with water conservation in mind. Unfortunately, xeriscaping has taken on a connotation of using rock, pebbles, and gravel to replace plants altogether. While the use of hard surfaces is a form of xeriscaping, it is not the only form. You can have a lush, beautiful landscape with much less water use without looking like you live on a rock quarry.

Regardless of what types of plants you use to xeriscape, the ones that you choose will not only need very little water, but they will also likely need very little care. Plants that can survive on exceptionally small amounts of water typically do not need large amounts of fertilizers and pruning to stay healthy and grow well. After all, these plants can survive in the wilderness with no care, so they should be fine in your yard. Research xeriscaping in your area to find out what plants will survive in your geographic zone.

Ditch the Lawn

The less lawn that you have to take care of, the less mowing and maintenance that you will have. It is that simple. You do not have to completely get rid of every patch of grass that you have to create a more maintenance-free landscape, but every little bit helps.

FACT

More than 60,000 severe accidents result from using lawn mowers each year. Twenty-five billion dollars are spent on the lawn care industry annually, while more than 580 million gallons of gas are used to run gas-powered lawn mowers. Up to 60 percent of a city's fresh water is used watering lawns, depending on the area.

You can eliminate grass but keep a lush green look by using low-growing ground covers, such as some jasmines, sedum, juniper, moss, dwarf mondo grass, or wooly thyme. Ask your local garden center what will work in your area. You can also increase the size of the garden beds in your landscape to reduce the amount of grass that you have, adding perennial or annual greenery or flowers to add living beauty.

Of course, if you want to get rid of anything green altogether, you can install pebbles and rocks on walkways and in entertaining areas, or large stone pavers that create a focal point in your landscape. Play areas can be heavily mulched to create a softer surface underneath a swing set or sandbox. Just make sure that keeping these areas weed-free and properly maintained won't cause additional work or require the use of more weed killers.

Edible Plants

So you are spending all of this time, money, and sweat on taking care of your lawn and garden, but what are you getting out of it? Sure, it is probably pretty, but wouldn't you like all of your hard work to be rewarded a little more? By incorporating more edible plants into your landscape, not only can you have a beautiful garden, but you will also have a healthy source of fruits and vegetables.

You do not have to completely ditch the grass and put in a field of crops to have an edible garden. Far from it. There are plenty of beautiful plants that just happen to produce food, too. For instance, instead of planting a crape myrtle tree in the backyard, why not plant a lemon or lime tree instead? Both are beautiful and have flowers at certain times of the year, but citrus trees have the added benefits of fragrant blossoms and fruit that you can share with neighbors, coworkers, or a local food bank.

You might be surprised at the types of plants that you can use in your landscape that can be eaten. There are many flowers, such as pansies and nasturtiums, that are edible if you use organic lawn care techniques. Herbs such as rosemary, mint, and dill can be taken out of pots and used as greenery in the garden beds, although mint has a tendency to grow out of control if not taken care of regularly. Lettuce, spinach, cabbage, and kale grow quickly and have beautiful leaves. Swiss chard is especially dramatic, with vibrant stalks that often contain neon shades of red, pink, or yellow. Squash plants shoot out bright orange-yellow blossoms, while sweet potatoes have a vibrant lime green or dark purple trailing vine of foliage.

ESSENTIAL

For more information on how to incorporate edible plants into your lawn and garden, find a book that explains the process and what will work in your geographic area. Some suggestions are *The Edible Front Yard* by Ivette Soler, *Landscaping with Fruit* by Lee Reich, *Eat Your Yard!* by Nan Chase, and *Edible Landscaping* by Rosalind Creasy.

Using some edible plants in your landscape can supply you and your family with healthy, home-grown food that will cost much less than at the grocery store and you know exactly how it was grown. Not only do you get a beautiful landscape, but you can eat healthier foods and save money at the same time. What a win-win situation!

CHECKLIST FOR A HEALTHIER LAWN AND GARDEN

- ❑ Avoid the use of synthetic weed killers and fertilizers. The harsh chemicals in lawn care products are similar to pesticides. Reduce your toxic exposure by choosing more natural products.
- ❑ Pick weeds by hand, or use a pre-emergent to stop them from growing. Removing weeds manually is the best way to get rid of them without any harmful exposures.
- ❑ Coffee grounds, compost, and waste from your kitchen make great all natural fertilizers. Use the power of nature to turn waste items into valuable garden amendments.
- ❑ Avoid using gas-powered lawn equipment, and use proper precautions if you must use it. Exhaust from lawn equipment can be worse than that from a car, so reduce the amount that you inhale.
- ❑ Use electric and manual lawn equipment when possible. You don't have to worry about inhaling toxic fumes when you use lawn equipment not powered by gasoline.
- ❑ Hire companies that only use nontoxic and environmentally preferable equipment and products. Let someone else do all of the hard work by hiring a professional who uses methods that make sense to you.
- ❑ Use native plants in your landscape to reduce your workload and chemical dependency. Plants that are adapted to your weather and soil do not have to be pampered as much to survive.
- ❑ Consider adding more edible plants to your landscape. If you go through all of the hassle of taking care of your garden, wouldn't it be nice to receive something in return?

CHAPTER 18

Outdoor Living

Ah, the great outdoors! There is nothing like getting out and enjoying some fresh air and the wonders of nature in your own backyard. Whether your idea of relaxing is taking a dip in the pool or cooking up a juicy steak while kicking back on your deck, there are some things to keep in mind to make your backyard just as healthy as your home. Being outside does not mean that you are immune from common household problems.

Pools

A beloved summer staple, swimming pools can offer countless hours of fun and physical activity for everyone. From backyard pools to community pools in housing developments or parks, there are nearly 9 million pools in America that offer a great way to socialize and enjoy pleasant weather. You might think that chlorine is the biggest health offender in a traditional swimming pool, but there are some other factors to consider.

Health Problems of Pools

The two major health problems associated with pools are recreational water illnesses (RWIs) and chlorine exposure. RWIs have symptoms such as diarrhea and skin, ear, eye, and respiratory infections. If a pool is treated and disinfected properly, most germs that cause RWIs are killed pretty quickly. For instance, *E. coli* can be killed in less than sixty seconds in a properly controlled pool, while it takes around forty-five minutes to kill the parasite *Giardia*. If a pool is not disinfected properly, which is often the case, the germs can survive in the water and infect swimmers.

Cryptosporidium (crypto) is the leading cause of problems such as diarrhea, vomiting, headaches, and abdominal pain known as gastroenteritis that are transmitted in swimming pools. Crypto is resistant to chlorine, and it takes more than ten days to kill the parasite in a properly controlled pool. Crypto-related cases increased by more than 200 percent from 2004 to 2008.

QUESTION

How are RWIs introduced into pool water?
The disgusting answer is that they are transmitted by feces, but even if you do not see something of that nature floating in the pool, it does not mean that it is not there. On average, there is about 0.14 grams of residual feces left on a person's backside—not just kids—and it washes off when you are in a pool.

Chlorine exposure also causes some people health problems such as skin, eye, and respiratory irritation. The chlorine itself might be the problem, but so can the pH level of the water. If the pH level of a pool's water is not regulated between 7.2 and 7.8, skin and eye irritation can occur, too, regardless of chlorine levels.

Keeping Pools Healthy

Pool water can be healthy, safe, and a great place to relax and play. But there are certain steps that must be taken in order to create a safe aquatic environment. Chlorine levels and pH levels must be constantly monitored, and good hygiene and common sense should always be in practice. For extensive information on how to keep your pool safe, the Water Quality and Health Council (*www.healthypools.org*) and the Centers for Disease Control (*www.cdc.gov/healthywater/swimming*) have excellent resources.

The chlorine levels in a swimming pool should always be greater than 1 part per million (ppm). Levels between 2 and 4 ppm are preferable. Levels for pH should be between 7.2 and 7.8. The pool water should not be cloudy and should not have a strong chlorine smell, which can actually be an indication of an unhealthy pool. If the pool's floor or sides feel sticky or slimy when you run your hands or feet over them, that is another indication that the water is not as clean as it should, or could, be.

ESSENTIAL

You can test the pH and free chlorine levels in your pool water or a community pool for free by ordering a test kit at no charge (*http:// healthypools.org/freeteststrips*). When you have the answers, you can upload the information to the same website to compare the health of your pool to others across the nation.

Kiddie Pools

Big pools are not the only places where there can be a big problem, though. Small children can have fun in a pool in the backyard by using an inflatable or molded plastic kiddie pool. These portable pools are easy, inexpensive, and convenient for homeowners who do not have a built-in pool. But the small amounts of water and lack of heavy-duty disinfectant systems can cause problems when children start sharing these pools.

RWIs can still be spread in kiddie pools because there is no disinfectants or filtration system used in these types of pools. Small pools are generally filled with tap water from a garden hose, and unless an additional disinfectant is added, there is not enough germ-killing power in tap water to kill germs that are brought in by humans.

According to the CDC, children should not be allowed to use kiddie pools in child care programs or at schools because of the risk of spreading water borne illnesses in untreated pool water. Children of the same household using one pool generally do not have problems, because they are used to being around each other and their family's germs. When children from many different settings start using the same pool, though, the chance for health problems is greater.

If portable pools are not drained every day after use, they should be treated with a disinfectant or filtration system to keep them germ-free. Doses and methods of germ-killing in smaller pools can be tricky, though, so it is essential to contact a professional before trying to treat the problem on your own, such as simply dumping chlorine bleach in the water, because self-administering disinfectants can be unhealthy and risky.

Saltwater Pools

Do saltwater pools offer any better protection? The salt in saltwater pools will kill bacteria and germs just like chlorine, without exposure to the harsh chemical additive. Small amounts of chlorine will still be produced by the natural reaction between the water and salt, but you do not add large amounts of the chemical into the pool—a benefit for anyone trying to avoid large amounts of chemicals. Saltwater pools, no matter what the name suggests, are not necessarily salty-tasting like ocean water.

Hot Tubs

A bubbling hot tub can do wonders to ease aches and pains and to erase the troubles of a hectic day. But hot tubs often have more health risks than pools do.

Less Disinfecting Power

The hot temperatures of hot tub water means that disinfectants such as chlorine can break down much faster than the disinfectants used in pools. When the disinfectants disappear rapidly in hot tub water, there is less germ-killing power in the water unless disinfectants are added even more frequently. Adding to the problem is that there is usually less water in relation to the number of bathers in a hot tub, compared to a pool. Have you ever seen a hot tub completely packed with people sitting on all of the seats inside? It is a common occurrence to see a small hot tub with at least eight to ten people, either sitting in it or with their feet dangling in it, at a hotel, resort, or party.

Hot Tub Rash

While RWIs can be present in both pools and hot tubs, there is one RWI known as "hot tub rash" that is most often associated with hot tubs. Hot tub rash is actually a skin infection, the symptoms of which can include:

- Itchy skin that develops a red, bumpy rash
- A rash on skin that was covered by a swimsuit
- Hair follicles infected with pus-filled blisters

Hot tub rash often lasts for just a few days. Usually it clears up by itself, and you might be unaware of what has happened. If the rash does not disappear on its own, though, you will need to seek medical attention.

Legionnaires' Disease

Legionnaires' disease is another type of illness that can be transmitted easily in hot tubs. Caused by a bacteria called *Legionella*, Legionnaires' disease is an infection of the lungs that often resembles pneumonia. Up to 18,000 people are hospitalized with Legionnaires' disease each year, and because it is caused by a bacteria, antibiotics are often necessary to treat the illness.

Legionnaires' disease is common in hot tubs because the bacteria grow especially well in hot water. Exposure to the bacteria occurs when someone inhales water that contains the bacteria, such as the vapor that rises off of the surface of a hot tub.

Symptoms of Legionnaires' disease are similar to the symptoms for pneumonia, including fever, chills, cough, muscle aches, and headaches. Only a chest X-ray and other diagnostic tests can tell whether the *Legionella* bacteria is present.

Keeping Hot Tubs Healthy

The steps to keep a hot tub healthy are basically the same as keeping a pool healthy. Ideal chlorine levels are between 2 and 4 ppm, while pH levels should remain between 7.2 and 7.8. Because chlorine and other disinfectants disappear so rapidly in a hot tub, the levels must be checked constantly, even as much as hourly during times of high use. Hot tubs should never feel slimy inside or have a strong chlorine odor, which can signal a problem. Putting a cover over a hot tub when it is not in use can help reduce the amount of disinfectants that can escape in the water. To keep the water-to-bather ratio low, always follow the hot tub's recommended guidelines for the maximum amount of people.

Hazardous Materials in the Garage

The garage tends to be the graveyard for everything that we do not want in our house. Leftover cans of paint, solvents, glues, gasoline, oil, lawn chemicals, pool chemicals—you name it and it is in the garage. So what is the problem? All of those items you are trying to keep out of your home might be coming back inside anyway. You might even be setting your family up for a dangerous incident.

Inhaling Chemical Fumes

If you have an attached garage, with at least one wall of the garage sharing a wall with another room in your home, you might be surprised at what could be happening. The fumes and VOCs coming from toxic products in the garage can find a way into your home through the walls, the air vents, and even the exchange of air every time you open the door into the garage.

It is especially problematic for the room closest to the garage or attached to the same wall.

What if you do not have an attached garage? You can still have the same problem of poor indoor air every time you enter the detached building, but it might be worse if you have a shed or small garage that is not climate-controlled. High temperatures in the garage will cause chemicals to off-gas from products even faster, raising toxin levels.

Limit What You Store

To truly have a healthy garage, you must rethink the toxic and hazardous chemicals and supplies that you keep. The more hazardous products that you have anywhere in your home, even in the garage, the greater the chance that they will cause you or your family members harm. Why not get rid of leftover paints, cleaning solutions, hobby supplies, and other items that you know that you will never use? Buy nontoxic, eco-friendly versions of the products that you would normally keep in the garage, from paints and glues to cleaning supplies and lawn chemicals, to avoid toxic exposures.

ALERT

Paints, cleaners, pesticides, and other items that you remove from your garage likely qualify as hazardous waste. Contact your local waste management division for disposal regulations in your area and for a schedule of hazardous-waste collection. You can also search Earth911.com (*www.earth911.com*) for a recycling center near you that takes these items.

Taking Proper Precautions

Sometimes you have no choice but to store toxic ingredients, such as gas and oil for the lawn mower or paint stripper for a project that you are constantly working on. Even if the chemicals are not off-gassing into your indoor air, though, there is still a risk, and it might surprise you—they are fire hazards, as well. The U.S. Fire Administration suggests the following ways to keep hazardous materials safely stored at home:

- Store hazardous materials in their original containers. If the label is peeling off, reattach it with transparent tape.
- Use proper storage containers for flammables and combustibles; buy products with safety closures whenever possible.
- Store flammable products, such as gasoline, kerosene, propane gas, and paint thinner in containers away from the house.
- Never store flammables in direct sunlight or near an open flame.
- Store hazardous materials out of the reach of children and pets.

Poison Control

No matter how hard you try to create a safe environment, sometimes accidents happen. If you have any amount of poisonous or hazardous materials in your garage or in your home—and just about everyone does—it is wise to have the number for your poison control help lines available in a place where you can access them quickly.

FACT

In 2009, more than 90 percent of all reported human poison exposures happened in a person's own home. Most deaths due to poisoning occur in adults. Ninety-three percent of all poisoning deaths in 2009 were in people age twenty or older, with the highest amount happening in adults age forty to forty-nine.

The American Association of Poison Control Centers (*www.aapcc.org*) operates fifty-seven poison centers across the country, but they can all be accessed with just one phone number: (800) 222-1222. Calling the number will automatically route you to your area poison control center every hour of the day, every day of the week. A search engine for local poison control centers and resources (*www.aapcc.org/dnn/AAPCC/FindLocalPoison Centers.aspx*) can offer additional information that you might find useful when trying to poison-proof your home.

Humans are not the only ones who can be injured by what is stored in the garage. Pets are often the victims of toxic exposures from hazardous materials thought to be tucked away safely outside of the home. The Animal Poison Control Center, operated by the ASPCA, can be reached twenty-four hours a day, every day of the year, at (888) 426-4435. The ASPCA offers answers to common poisoning questions in pets in their "Animal Poison Control FAQ" (*www.aspca.org/pet-care/poison-control/animal-poison-control-faq.aspx*).

Decking and Play Sets

If you have any wooden structures in your backyard, such as a deck, railings, a play set, wooden walkways, etc., chances are the wood has been chemically treated with some type of pesticide. While redwood and cedar do not have to be treated because they have natural protective qualities, all other woods must have some type of artificial defense to protect from rot, fungi, and pests, which will destroy the wood in a matter of years. This is a serious concern; wooden backyard structures can have a lot of direct exposure with your skin, from walking barefoot across a deck to children playing on swing sets and putting their hands in their mouths while playing.

Chromated Copper Arsenate (CCA)

Have you ever seen a swing set or a deck made from wood that had a slightly greenish tint? That greenish color does not mean that the wood that was used to make those items was really new. It turns out that lumber with a greenish tint was likely preserved with arsenic-based chemicals, especially chromated copper arsenate (CCA). CCA was among the most widely used chemical used on pressure-treated wood from the 1970s to 2004. Arsenic-treated lumber usually had a greenish tint, but not always.

CCA, a chemical mixture that contains arsenic, chromium, and copper, was often used to protect wood from the pests, mold, and fungus problems common for products used outside. Since CCA is designed to kill living organisms, such as mold, it is a registered pesticide. One of the ingredients of CCA, arsenic, is a known carcinogen, and is known to cause health problems such as nerve damage, dizziness, numbness, and immune diseases.

In 2003, the wood industry voluntarily discontinued the use of CCA in pressure-treated wood used for residential uses. As of December 30, 2003,

CCA-treated lumber cannot be used for most items in residential settings, including play structures, picnic tables, fencing, decking, timber used for landscaping, boardwalks, and patios. There has never been an official ban on CCA-pressure-treated wood by the CPSC because of the voluntary recall.

FACT

An area of wood the size of a four-year-old's hand, if treated with arsenic, contains 120 times more arsenic than allowed by the EPA in a six-ounce glass of water. Soil below wood decks that have been treated with CCA had arsenic concentrations that were elevated by 2,000 percent.

Though CCA-treated wood is not used in homes anymore, it can still be used in other places where you spend time and are exposed to the chemical. Wood treated with CCA is still allowed to be used in commercial settings, such as materials for fence posts and structural support, as well as certain residential uses such as shingles and structural items other than decks.

Pressure-Treated Woods

While CCA has been banned from use in most residential uses, that does not mean that other chemicals are not being used in its place. Preservatives such as cyproconazole, propiconazole, ACQ, and copper azole are just being used in its place. While the arsenic in CCA is known to cause cancer, there are many new types of wood preservatives that are still not widely understood. The EPA says that because "ACQ and copper azole have been developed relatively recently and/or have been used infrequently, only limited research has been conducted on their potential leaching and environmental impact."

If you want to use pressure-treated wood, one of the most well-researched and least-toxic alternatives is to use preservatives made from borate, such as disodium octoborate tetrahydrate (DOT). Borates are minerals that can be found in nature in all living things and have a minimal impact on the environment. In order to have pressure-treated wood treated with borate preservatives, you will need to specially request it from your home contractor or ask for it specifically at the lumber store.

Wondering how you can avoid pesticide-treated materials in your backyard and still be able to enjoy the great outdoors? The EPA's "Chromated Copper Arsenate (CCA): Alternatives to Pressure-Treated Wood" (*www.epa.gov/oppad001/reregistration/cca/pressuretreated-wood_alternatives.htm*) offers suggestions of a wide array of building materials, including woods, composites, and plastics, as well as their advantages and disadvantages.

Protect Yourself from Exposure

If you have CCA-treated wood at home, it is up to you to protect yourself from arsenic exposure. According to the CPSC, "The voluntary cancellations did not address the potential exposure to chemical residues from existing CCA-wood structures, nor does the EPA require the removal of structures made with CCA-treated wood." So just because CCA-treated wood is not sold anymore, that does not mean that you are protected from its toxic effects. To be safe, you should follow some guidelines to reduce your risk, not just at home, but also on any public structures, such as playgrounds, picnic tables, and boardwalks at places such as schools, parks, and apartment buildings. Assume that all wood outdoors has been treated with some type of preservative, whether CCA or not.

Always make sure that you and other members of your family wash your hands after touching wood that could have been pressure-treated with arsenic, whether after playing on a play set or just grasping the hand rail of a deck. Use a tablecloth on picnic tables that might be made of arsenic-treated wood, whether at home or at parks, and never lay any type of food directly on pressure-treated wood.

Do not allow children and pets to play in soil that might be contaminated from pressure-treated lumber, such as a dirt mound located underneath elevated decking made from arsenic-treated lumber. Never use CCA-treated wood in structures used to grow vegetables or any other type of edible plant, such as in raised garden beds or planters made of CCA-treated wood. If CCA-treated wood had been used in an area where food is being grown, consider replacing the topsoil and adding a few inches of fresh soil to the area.

ALERT

If you cannot remove arsenic-treated wood structures at your home, try sealing the wood every six months with a penetrating deck treatment, which might help reduce your exposure to chemicals. But do not use deck washes on CCA-treated wood because certain chemicals in these products can cause even more problems in conjunction with the arsenic. Power washing CCA-treated wood can also cause exposure to the chemicals, too, so it is important to always think about and research your cleaning options if you think that you have CCA-treated wood decks.

Removal of Pressure-Treated Woods

When it comes time to remove pressure-treated wood, removal should be done with great caution. Whether you or a professional removes the wood, try to avoid creating sawdust. Chances are there will be some sawdust and small chips of the wood that are created, so be sure to wear goggles, a dust mask, and gloves, and take proper precautions during the entire process. Clean up as much of the debris from the wood as you can and properly dispose of it. These shavings and sawdust should not be allowed to be disposed of elsewhere on your property to naturally decompose. If you cannot replace an entire arsenic-treated wooden structure, consider just replacing the areas where there is constant contact, such as handrails, exposed deck planks, etc.

Since arsenic, and any other chemicals, can leach into the soil, it is wise to remove the top 2 to 5 inches of topsoil underneath a structure containing arsenic and dispose of them properly, since arsenic will not biodegrade or disappear on its own.

Never burn any pressure-treated wood, regardless of whether it was treated with CCA or not. The chemicals that are used in the wood are released into the smoke and inhaled.

CHECKLIST FOR A HEALTHY BACKYARD

❑ Store hazardous materials properly. Many household injuries and poisonings are due to accidental exposure to toxic materials commonly found in the home. Prevent the problems in the first place by limiting access to anything that could be dangerous to members of your family.

❑ Always wash hands after touching pressure-treated wood. Toxic chemicals can rub off onto your skin, which can then be absorbed or ingested.

❑ Constantly monitor a pool for proper chlorine levels and pH balance to prevent the spread of infection. Germs can be killed in a pool, but only if the water is properly treated each and every day.

❑ Hot tubs require extra maintenance and monitoring of chlorine and pH levels to curb bacterial growth. The warm temperatures of hot tub water create a breeding ground for pathogens.

❑ Reduce the amount of hazardous materials that you keep at home. The fewer toxins you have at home, the less risk you have of unhealthy exposure to them.

❑ Do not grow food or allow children or pets to play in soil that has been exposed to pressure-treated wood. Arsenic residues can remain in soil even when the wood is no longer present.

❑ Never burn pressure-treated wood. Chemicals used in preserving wood will be released into smoke, which can then be inhaled.

CHAPTER 19

At Work

No matter where you work, whether it is a home office, a cubicle in a major international company, or a table at the local coffeehouse, your work environment can affect your health. Sometimes you can be in direct control of your work environment. Other times you have to go to work regardless of how unhealthy the building might be. Considering you spend the majority of your day working, it is important to try to create a healthy work environment just as you would create a healthy home.

Electronics

Chances are you deal with some kind of electronic product at work, from computers to scanners to a copy machine. The act of processing and sending information can not only tax your brain, but it can also be problematic to your health.

Fire Retardants

Fire retardants are most often associated with mattresses and textiles, but electronic equipment needs fire retardants, too, because of the heat that can be produced. Just as fire-retardant exposure can be a concern with bedding materials, there is also concern about exposure to toxic fire retardants through electronic equipment.

One fire retardant in particular, known as deca, is often used in electronics, especially television and computer monitors. Deca is just one type of fire retardant in a group of chemical fire retardants known as PBDEs, which are now the subject of intense scrutiny because of their toxic effects in the environment and potentially on human health. Deca is thought to possibly cause cancer and affect brain function.

ALERT

Just because U.S. manufacturers must stop using deca by 2013, that does not mean that your computer might be deca-free. Imported electronics are not held to the same ban. Older electronics manufactured before 2013 can still contain deca, as well as other fire retardants.

The chemical deca has been found in very high levels in Californians, probably because products in their state have to meet extremely high fire-resistance levels where as other states do not require the same flammability standards. With an increase of these PBDE chemicals being found in humans, many people are demanding that PBDEs should stop being used. In fact, federal law will now require U.S. manufacturers to stop using deca by the year 2013.

Laptops

Laptop computers are supposed to be convenient because they can be used while sitting on—not surprisingly—your lap. It turns out, though, that the added convenience of laptop computing could actually be affecting the fertility of men around the world.

In a study published in the journal *Fertility and Sterility*, researchers discovered that the temperature of men's scrotums heated very rapidly when they were working with a laptop on their knees. It is thought that when the scrotum is heated, even by just a couple of degrees, that sperm are affected in an adverse way. The study found that a laptop heated the scrotum by more than four degrees in one hour, though unsafe temperatures started occurring within fifteen minutes.

Pillows and lap pads did not offer any temperature protection, either. The best way to avoid possible overheating of any body part is to use the laptop on a table.

Work Locations

Creating a healthy work environment is directly related to where and how you work. Sometimes the process can be extremely easy; perhaps it is not even an issue. Other times, you might feel as if you have no say in fixing the problems that you know are causing health problems for you and others.

Self-Employed or Working From Home

If you work from home, either telecommuting for a company or because you are self-employed, you have wonderful access to creating a healthy work environment. Making sure that your office is healthy is no different from making sure that the rest of your home is healthy. You can control the office equipment that you buy, as well as the indoor air quality.

If you own a company where you and other workers are employed, you are directly responsible for ensuring that your employees are working in a healthy environment. If there are problems, you have the authority to fix them. You can set standards that ensure a nontoxic work setting for everyone. Should there be a structural problem with your location that has serious health consequences, you are the one to decide how to fix it and whether you need to move.

Working at the Office

If you work for someone else and must go to a workplace every day, your control over your work environment can be extremely limited. You might be lucky enough to work for a boss or company that is committed to creating a healthy work environment for everyone and takes care of problems when they occur. Or you might work in a place with known health hazards that management is not taking seriously. It can be challenging to work in a place where someone else is making the decisions about what a "healthy" environment means.

The Most Common Workplace Offender

Poor indoor air quality is by far the most common workplace health hazard. Regardless of what type of work that you do, from office work to processing materials in a factory, the lack of fresh air in a workplace can cause health problems. Fixing the problem is not as easy as making the air-conditioning system run more. Indoor air in a work location is very complicated and might not be easily fixed.

Pollutants in Indoor Air

An office building's air can become heavily polluted just by the simple day-to-day activities that occur. Many different people come to work each day, whether just a handful of employees at a small company or hundreds of individuals in a large corporation. Each person brings a unique set of germs and viruses, perfumes and scented personal care products, lingering tobacco smoke odors, and more.

The machines, products, and building materials of a work environment also contribute to indoor pollutants. Copy machines, scanners, and toners can release fumes. Cleaners and pesticides that are used indoors can build up in the indoor air. Building materials off-gas chemicals for years after construction. The sheer volume of desks, chairs, bookcases, and other office furniture can mean that there are high levels of formaldehyde and other chemicals floating around in the air.

ALERT

Even just the amount of carbon dioxide that people give off during the course of a day can contribute to poor indoor air quality and cause health problems. If the levels of carbon dioxide are allowed to build up, it can contribute to headaches and feelings of drowsiness, which results in less work being able to be done.

Mold is another common indoor air pollutant, especially in older buildings that might have had plumbing leaks and other moisture problems. Mold can be hidden behind the walls and never seen or smelled, so it can be hard to determine that mold is causing a problem. In other offices, however, workers can actually see mold growing on ceiling tiles or on walls and along floorboards.

Lack of Ventilation

Poor indoor air quality occurs when there is a lack of ventilation. Ventilation does not only mean air flowing within a building, such as when the air-conditioning or heating system might be on. Air movement from a vent does not indicate proper ventilation.

Ventilation for healthy indoor air means removing the existing indoor air, full of the pollutants, and exchanging it for fresher air, which most often comes from outside. It is not enough to simply recirculate indoor air that is contaminated. The required levels of ventilation have decreased for new buildings, because of concern over energy use. It costs a lot of money to heat cold air during the winter or to cool hot air during the summer, so the amount of outdoor air that is required for ventilation systems is lower than in years and decades past.

While there are standards for how much fresh air is needed for a building's ventilation system, keep in mind that those standards are just for when the building is built. That does not mean that the ventilation system of a building is actually operating at those standards. Problems with a ventilation system, altering the outdoor air intake, or turning off the system means that the minimum ventilation standards, which are already low, may not be reached.

In the quest to save energy and reduce heating and cooling bills, building operators might actually be causing more problems than they are preventing. Turning off a ventilation system when there are no occupants in the building, such as at night and on weekends, allows the indoor air pollutants to rise to high levels before the system turns back on. Even just reducing the ventilation when a room is not occupied, rather than turning it off, can also cause problems. Ventilation not only removes pollutants, but it also controls humidity levels. When humidity is allowed to increase in a building, mold starts to grow and soon becomes another indoor air pollutant that can cause health problems and must be fixed.

Sick Building Syndrome

Sick building syndrome (SBS) can be a problem with any type of building, including your home. But SBS is most often associated with office buildings and work environments. The World Health Organization believes that nearly one-third of new and remodeled buildings have unusually high complaints of symptoms associated with SBS.

SBS cannot be diagnosed with a medical test. The illness is characterized by physical symptoms that do not have a cause that can be definitively identified. Symptoms can include eye, nose, and throat irritation, headaches, and fatigue. One of the leading factors in diagnosing SBS is that a person feels physically better after they have left the building.

SBS is thought to be linked with poor indoor air quality. When indoor air is not ventilated properly, contaminants can start to build up. Those contaminants, whether chemical or natural in nature, can cause health problems.

In a study published in the journal *Occupational and Environmental Medicine*, symptoms of SBS decreased significantly when indoor air quality was improved. Forty to fifty percent of workers had fewer symptoms of SBS six months after the ventilation system of their office was improved. Three years later, the levels of SBS symptoms were still low compared to the office workers' complaints before the new ventilation system was installed.

What You Can Do

It might seem frustrating that you do not have more say in how healthy that your work environment is, but you actually have more influence than you might think. Your actions, and the actions of your coworkers, can dramatically affect the health and quality of your workplace away from home.

Improving the Indoor Air

The EPA offers guidelines on the steps that office workers can take to prevent indoor air quality problems, including:

- Do not block air vents or grilles. Perhaps your office is freezing and you are tired of wearing a sweater, so you block off an air vent. Or maybe a filing cabinet has been placed in front of an air grille. The less ventilation that occurs in a building, even with just an air vent closed, means less reduction of pollutants from the indoor air.
- Abide by office smoking policies. Smoke only in designated areas. If outdoor smoke is coming into the building, designate smoking areas farther away from the doors and entryways.
- Clean up spills quickly and report leaks immediately. Moisture creates mold problems. If leaks and spills are not dried and removed quickly, mold and fungus can become a problem.
- Dispose of garbage. Things in the garbage can create foul odors and bacterial growth. Remove the garbage often and only allow trash to be thrown out in designated areas.
- Store foods properly. Rotting food can cause odors and health problems. Food can also attract pests, which means the need for pesticides. Clean up food spills, keep the refrigerator clean and tidy, and

wash communal dishes, cups, and silverware often to prevent the spread of health problems.

- Notify the building manager if you suspect an indoor air quality problem.

Add Some Plants

Adding houseplants to indoors has been proven to improve indoor air quality and remove pollutants such as formaldehyde and benzene from the air. Houseplants can help to naturally purify the air of your office environment just as they do in your home.

Not only do plants help improve indoor air quality, but they can also improve the way that you function while at work. A study in *HortScience* found that people are generally happier when they work with plants in the office environment. The research participants felt better about their jobs and their work and rated their job satisfaction and quality of life higher. They even were more positive about their bosses and coworkers.

Even if you do not have any windows in your office environment, you can still find a plant that will grow. Thankfully, some of the toughest plants that can survive in low-light conditions, even with just artificial office lights, are also the ones that can remove the most pollutants. These plants can also be extremely tolerant of lack of watering and other common abuses by people who were born without green thumbs. Among the most effective plants at removing toxins from the air are:

- Areca palm
- Peace lily
- Rubber plant
- Weeping fig
- Dracaena
- English ivy
- Boston fern
- Spider plant

Adding just one or two plants to your desk can help improve the indoor air in your immediate area. For even more air filtration, ask if you or your company can add plants throughout the work area, such as in the kitchen and other common areas, along walkways, or in the lobby. One plant can clean about 100 square feet of air, so the more plants that there are that have demonstrated air filtering properties, the cleaner the air will be.

FACT

All plants will absorb the carbon dioxide that people exhale in their breath. In exchange, plants release oxygen that people need for healthy air. The buildup of carbon dioxide from many people in an office can cause low levels of productivity. Plants naturally will absorb that carbon dioxide.

Bring an Air Filter

Maybe you can't have plants in your office for a variety of reasons. That does not mean that you can't find another way to filter the air around you. There are many versions of tabletop mechanical air filters that are designed for use in an office environment. As long as you have an electrical outlet nearby, you can plug in a small air filter to clean the air in your immediate vicinity. Personal air filters will not work to clean the entire office environment, and might not make a dramatic difference if there are serious problems affecting your office's indoor air quality. But every little bit helps, and many people who use personal air filter systems report a reduction in the symptoms that can be caused by indoor air. Just be sure to clean the air filter regularly, whether by replacing or washing the filter, and look for one that removes the smallest size of microns and can clean the largest amount of air.

Fighting for a Healthier Work Environment

There are many steps you and your coworkers can take to create a healthier workplace. Sometimes those steps are just not enough. Whether you are trying to fix the problems alone or there are larger problems that are out of your control, perhaps you just are not making any positive changes in your building's quality of health and therefore your health is suffering. There are still actions that you can take so that you, and everyone who works in your building, can be protected from health hazards.

FACT

The total cost of lost productivity and work because of employees calling in sick can be more than $63 billion each year. More than 4,000 people miss either work or school each day because of asthma-related problems, which can be exacerbated by poor indoor air. Asthma is the fourth leading cause of missing work, according to the Asthma and Allergy Foundation of America.

Ask Around

You might not be the only person who is having health problems because of something in the workplace. Most people do not sit around and talk about all of their aches and pains (although you probably know a few that do). Just because people are not talking about it does not mean that they are not experiencing any problems, though. The more people who are having physical problems caused by the workplace, then the more likely you are to get the problem fixed.

Perhaps someone is having symptoms, but has not associated them with the office. Or maybe there is a definite relation to a change at work and an increase in health problems, such as more people having allergies after new carpeting was installed, or more coworkers with asthma who experienced flareups after a room was painted.

Talk to the Bosses

Do not assume that your boss or management has any idea that there might be a health problem in the office or workplace. Perhaps they do not spend the same amount of time that you do in the building. Or maybe they are just too concerned with management issues to have even considered workplace health hazards. Whatever the reason, it is unwise to accuse your boss of allowing health problems to occur.

When meeting with your superiors, or whoever might be the person to talk to about health concerns, speak calmly. Give a matter-of-fact description of the symptoms that you and other coworkers are experiencing, and what you think that might be the cause. If you do not have an idea of what could be causing the symptoms, that is okay. Reporting that they are happening is the first step in finding out what the problem is.

Your boss might immediately agree that there could be a problem, or maybe they will be skeptical and dismiss your claims, especially if the symptoms are vague and cannot be directly contributed to a specific occurrence or product. Either way, it is necessary to report the problems to get anything done. Before ending the conversation, ask what the next step should be. Your boss might just want you to monitor your symptoms for a longer period of time to see if they continue. You might need to report the problem to a different person in the company, fill out a special form, or file a formal complaint before anything can be done. Ideally, management will fix the problem immediately to prevent any future health problems in employees.

Report Problems

To document how your workplace might be making you sick, you need to report your symptoms to the appropriate people. First, start writing down the specifics for your own records and for future talks with medical professionals. Keep track of points such as:

- When did you first start noticing the symptoms?
- Do your symptoms improve when you leave work at the end of the day?
- Do your symptoms improve in a short period of time, such as when you leave the building on your lunch break?
- Can your symptoms be linked to a specific event, such as after the building was flooded by a burst pipe or after a renovation?
- Have your symptoms been getting worse?
- What makes your symptoms go away?
- What other tests and what other doctors have you gone to in order to rule out other causes? What have been the treatments that they offered you, and did they work?

Next, visit a medical professional. For large corporations, you might have a medical person on staff or a company-sponsored clinic. You can also visit your personal physician, who knows your medical history and whether these symptoms are new and unusual. In certain cases, when an action occurred at work caused you harm, you might file a worker's compensation claim, and you will need to go to assigned doctors that handle worker's compensation visits. Every situation is different, yet there is always someone to whom you should talk about your health problems.

Having a file of health problems that could be caused by your work environment will make it much easier to encourage the company to make the appropriate changes. It also can assist investigators in health and safety standards investigations, if needed, and supports your claim if you should ever need to file legal action or receive medical benefits. Doctors' notes can also be valuable leverage in encouraging management to implement healthy changes in the office that will benefit the health of everyone.

CHECKLIST FOR A HEALTHY WORK ENVIRONMENT

- ❏ Talk about your concerns about poor indoor air quality with the appropriate individuals. Poor indoor air is among the most common health complaints in workplace settings, and causes many sick days among employees. If you think that there is a problem, bring it up with someone who can remedy the situation.
- ❏ Use a tabletop mechanical air filter to reduce indoor air pollutants. To clean the air in your part of the workplace, an air filter can help remove some of the problems.
- ❏ Bring a plant or two into the office for natural air cleaning power. Some plants will actually absorb common chemicals and help purify the air naturally.
- ❏ Do not balance a laptop on your lap; use a table instead. High levels of heat can build up around your reproductive organs, even though you do not feel an increase in temperature.
- ❏ Do not block air vents in the office, which can lead to improper ventilation. Fresh air cannot get into your workplace if the vents are blocked.
- ❏ Keep a record of your health symptoms, and report them to medical professionals. If you believe that your workplace is contributing to health problems, keep detailed reports for future needs.

CHAPTER 20

Encouraging a Healthy School

Outside of your home, your children spend most of their time at school. If you work hard to reduce and eliminate toxic exposures at home, you do not want all of your hard work to be undone by an unhealthy school environment. There are a variety of ways to encourage your child's school to take action to create a healthier learning environment not just for your child, but for all children.

Lack of Regulation

After going through your house room by room and learning what the potential toxins are that can affect your family's health, you might be a little shocked at the dangers that are allowed to be present in a person's home. A house is not the only place where these toxins could be lurking, though. In fact, the place where you and other parents send their children to school all day is probably not as healthy as you might think.

FACT

> In 2010, more than 49 million students attended public elementary and secondary schools, with an additional one million attending public prekindergarten, according to the National Center for Education Statistics. Approximately 5.8 million students attended private prekindergarten, elementary, and secondary schools, according to the Council for American Private Education. Throughout both public and private schools, 6 million staff members work each day.

Get ready, because this quote might shock you. According to the Coalition for Healthier Schools' "Sick Schools 2009" report, "no outside public health or environment agency is responsible for providing effective enforcement, protections, or interventions specifically for schoolchildren at risk or suffering from the effects of poor air quality, chemical mismanagement and spills, or other hazards." Yes, you did read that correctly. When it comes to keeping your children safe from environmental hazards within a school, there is little regulation.

Among the nation's public schools, more than two out of every three schools have an infrastructure problem such as a leaking roof, which could potentially cause environmental health hazards. More than half of all public schools have at least one unsatisfactory environmental factor. Yet with all of the health risks affecting more than 98 percent of all schoolchildren each year, the EPA, the CDC, and many other government agencies do not have any authority to enter a school and determine whether children's health is affected by an environmental cause.

Environmental Hazards

The same environmental hazards that are common at home are usually common throughout a school. Many school buildings are very old and in need of repair, which only exacerbates environmental problems. Unless your school or school system specifically looks for these health hazards, they might be overlooked.

Pesticides

Pesticides can cause a variety of health problems, from dizziness, headaches, and rashes to asthma and cancer. Children are most vulnerable to toxic pesticide exposure because their bodies are still rapidly developing. Ironically, even though children are so susceptible to pesticides, they are commonly and extensively used in many schools throughout the year.

FACT

According to Beyond Pesticides (*www.beyondpesticides.org*), among forty commonly used pesticides in schools, twenty-eight can cause cancer, fourteen are linked to endocrine disruption, twenty-six have been shown to adversely affect reproduction, twenty-six damage the nervous system, and thirteen can cause birth defects.

You might think limiting your child's exposure to pesticides will be an uphill battle. The good news is, though, that many school systems have recognized the risk and have implemented policies to help reduce pesticide exposure. State governments can create stricter school pesticide policies that limit every child's exposure at school. Local school districts can implement stricter standards, too. Not every state has created a school pesticide policy, but more than two-thirds of the nation's states have enacted guidelines that either use integrated pest management, pesticide bans, or right-to-know policies in which parents and caregivers must be informed prior to any pesticide application. A list of states and school districts that have pesticide policies and programs (*www.beyondpesticides.org/schools/school policies/index.htm*) can be researched on Beyond Pesticides' website.

Just because your state or local school district has a pesticide policy does not mean that the children are not at risk from pesticide exposure, though. It simply means that there are guidelines in place regarding pesticide use. For instance, the state of New York has a policy that parents, guardians, and staff who have registered with the school will receive notice forty-eight hours in advance of a pesticide application, though pesticides will still be used. At Denver and Boulder Valley, Colorado, school districts, however, using integrated pest management curbed a mice problem without the use of pesticides.

If you are concerned about pesticide use at your child's school but don't know how to approach the school, there are plenty of resources available online. A great place to start is with information from the School Pesticide Reform Coalition (*www.beyondpesticides.org/toxicfreeschools/whatyou cando.htm*). You can quickly and easily download a postcard (*www .beyondpesticides.org/toxicfreeschools/index.htm*) that you and fellow parents can send to school officials highlighting the risk of pesticide use and asthma in children. If you are interested in organizing a safer pest management program at school, you can print off a pamphlet (*www.beyond pesticides.org/schools/publications/school_organizing.pdf*) that will tell you all of the information that you need.

Poor Indoor Air Quality

"Children miss school every day because of illnesses triggered by indoor air pollutants," said Amy Garcia, the former executive director of the National Association of School Nurses. Poor indoor air quality can lead to many health problems, most notably asthma, which is a serious problem among schools. With nearly one out of every eight children in school having asthma, resulting in nearly 15 million school days missed each year, poor indoor air quality and its effect on asthma is a very real and serious concern for schoolchildren and their parents. Poor indoor air quality is such a concern because it is so widely prevalent, yet so easily preventable. The EPA estimated that nearly 50 percent of all schools have indoor air problems.

The EPA has created an IAQ Tools for Schools Kit, which helps schools improve their indoor air quality (IAQ) with low- or no-cost methods. The kit shows schools how to use their own staff to implement changes to improve the entire school's indoor air. Most of the information can be downloaded by schools for free (*www.epa.gov/iaq/schools/actionkit.html#Order*). Schools can also request a free IAQ Problem Solving Wheel and video collection, as well as the kit on CD-ROM, on the same website. The Healthy Schools Network's handy checklist (*www.nationalhealthyschoolsday.org/mediaKit/Healthly_Indoor_Air_Checklist.pdf*) can also help your child's school check the quality of their indoor air.

Mold

Mold is just one of the many problems leading to poor indoor air within schools. Water leaks that are not taken care of quickly or properly can lead to the growth of mold. Mold can lurk unseen for years in walls and ceilings, but the health effects can definitely be felt. Carpets can harbor mold if there has been a water leak since the carpeting has been installed. Even lack of ventilation and climate control can lead to serious mold problems, such as when air-conditioning in a building is turned off over the weekend or on school holidays to save money. In one Orlando, Florida, school, where mold was clearly visible on the walls and floor, the humidity levels were found to be approximately 86 percent, an ideal breeding ground for mold.

Cleaners

Harsh chemical cleaners can also be a major cause of poor indoor air quality. In the quest to keep schools clean, a variety of disinfectants, window cleaners, floor cleaners, and room deodorizers are used in every room of the school. If these cleaners are full of toxic chemicals, the chemicals will continue to build up in the indoor air. If there is a lack of ventilation within the school, the problem is especially serious because the chemical buildup will not easily disappear and be replaced with fresh air. It does not take chemicals to keep a school clean and germ-free. Quality green cleaners that are nontoxic and do not contribute to poor indoor air quality have been found to be just as effective and easily available to school systems. The entire state of Illinois has even mandated that green cleaners be used in all public and private elementary and secondary schools with more than fifty students.

FACT

Two schools in Honolulu, Hawaii, were able to slash their cleaning product expenditure from $6 to $12 per gallon for conventional restroom cleaning products to less than $1 per gallon. The cost savings came when the schools started using a concentrated Green Seal–certified product, a widely respected certification for healthier, more sustainable products.

Want to encourage your child's school to switch to greener cleaners? The EWG (*www.ewg.org/schoolcleaningsupplies/faq*) offers tips on talking to schools to ask that they use green cleaning products. The same website also has a letter that can be customized by you to send to school officials, as well as a fact sheet about certified green cleaning supplies that can be included in the mailing. Cleaning for Healthy Schools (*www.cleaning forhealthyschools.org*) has great advice on ways to approach a school system to request that they use green cleaners. On the website you will find customizable presentations and handouts, as well as a poster on green cleaning health benefits by the National Association of School Nurses.

Water Quality

The Safe Drinking Water Act (SDWA) strives to regulate the amount of toxins or contaminants that are allowed to be present in the nation's public drinking water supply. The water coming into your school might be safe from the source. But lead pipes within the school could be corroding and adding toxic lead to the water that would not show up in your city or town's water quality reports. Lead in school's drinking water is such a concern that the EPA discusses it extensively on its website (*http://water.epa.gov/drink/ info/lead/schools_index.cfm*). The resources include the common problems and health risks specifically for schools. The only way to measure the lead level of the water at your child's school is to test the water coming out of the faucet directly at the school. The EPA has also created guidelines (*http:// water.epa.gov/drink/info/lead/testing.cfm*) specifically to help schools test their drinking water for lead.

If a school has a well, the problem is more common, according to an Associated Press (AP) investigation in 2009. Using data from the EPA, the AP discovered that nearly one out of every five schools with a well had violated the SDWA in the past decade. Though it is required for schools with wells to test their water, the chain of government paperwork means that some violations are never adequately reported or even recognized.

ALERT

If a school's water supply is not regulated by the SDWA, it does not mean that the water quality is necessarily bad. It is the responsibility of each water system to test its own water for health and safety standards. If there are no concerns present, or if the water system appropriately handles those concerns, the water should not pose a threat.

Shockingly, the EPA estimates that approximately 90,000 public elementary and secondary schools are not under the regulations of the SDWA. Schools that are not regulated by the SDWA may or may not be voluntarily testing their water. Though contaminated water is a very real concern, and is especially problematic for children, the EPA does not have authority to test water in schools.

Parental Support

If you are upset about the potential health risks at your child's school, chances are there are other parents who feel the same way. Some parents and guardians might already be aware of the dangers, but many are probably not even aware of the risks. The more people who are disturbed about the health hazards at a school and want a positive change, the more likely it is that an individual school, school district, or even state government will take action.

Your first step in gaining parental support is simply to educate parents about the possible health risks at your child's school. Do not assume that everyone knows that pesticides or mold can lead to asthma, or that lead could be in the water and contributing to problems in learning at school. These are health topics that are not talked about often, and many parents might just assume that there are strict standards in place to protect their children while they spend their days at school.

Try to find a nonthreatening way to educate parents about these health dangers and encourage them to take action with you. Use your existing social networks to gather parents together to learn about and discuss the problems. Have a potluck dinner and invite a local medical expert to come and talk about toxic health risks at school. Ask if you can insert an article in a newsletter or send an e-mail to children's parents. Talk with other parents and guardians who attend the school's PTA meetings or local government events. Start a Facebook page where parents can learn about health risks and positive actions whenever it is convenient for them to go online. Start a petition asking for a specific change in your school. Don't ask parents to support new policies that they might not understand. Parents who are educated about the problems and see the risks are more apt to join you in the fight for healthier schools.

The Healthy Schools Network (*www.healthyschools.org*) has a wide array of resources such as pamphlets, posters, and videos available that can guide you through the process of encouraging your child's school to become healthier. The organization sponsors a National Healthy Schools Day each year (*www.nationalhealthyschoolsday.org*), which is sponsored by the EPA, CDC, and many other health organizations. This national event is an ideal time to hold an event and partner with other schools across the country to raise awareness among parents and administration.

Talking to Teachers

Your children are not the only ones who can be affected by toxic health risks at a school. The teachers and staff who work in the school are exposed to the same dangers. Approaching the teachers and staff as allies in the fight for a healthier school encourages a less-toxic environment for everyone who spends most of their days in the building.

Your child's teachers could be your best liaison in your quest to create a nontoxic school. After all, the teachers are with your child each and every day. As adults, they can recognize potentially unhealthy situations and products better than your children. They might be aware of changes in your child's health or cognitive abilities in conjunction with certain activities at school. The teachers also have a more direct line of communication with the school staff and administration than many parents.

Get to Know the Teachers

Getting to know your child's teacher, and creating a relationship in which you are both striving toward what is best for your child and his education, is absolutely necessary in partnering with a teacher to create a healthier school. Take every opportunity to talk with the teacher during parent-teacher meetings or other events that the school organizes. Ask how you can stay in touch with the teacher during the year should you have any concerns. Invite your child's teachers to any parent meeting that you have regarding health risks at schools. Teachers need to be educated about the potential health risks in school just like parents and guardians. Keep in mind, though, that your child's teacher is there to educate your child at school, not to make policy changes. They might be just as frustrated as you are with the system. But as more people become concerned with a school's health, changes are more likely to occur.

Teaching Environmental Health

Perhaps you could encourage your child's teachers to incorporate topics about environmental health concerns into their curriculum when possible. There are many resources available that will not only educate teachers and their students, but might also end up educating more parents and the school administration. The EPA has a wealth of resources (*www.epa.gov/students/teachers.html*). There are also curriculum plans at The National Institute of Environmental Health Sciences (*www.niehs.nih.gov/health/scied/*), the National Library of Medicine's Tox Town (*http://toxtown.nlm.nih.gov/text_version/teachers.php*), and the State of Washington's Department of Ecology Hazards on the Homefront Teacher's Guides (*www.ecy.wa.gov/hazardson thehomefront/index.html*).

Suggest Alternatives

Perhaps you know what the potential health hazards are at your child's school. You have gained support from fellow parents and teachers who want things to change. Now is the time to approach the school administration or school system and ask for healthier standards for your child's school.

Be Specific

When requesting changes be made to a school to reduce health risks, it always easier to ask for something specific rather than something vague. For instance, instead of asking for an improvement in the indoor air quality of your child's school, specifically ask that plumbing leaks be fixed immediately to prevent mold from growing and that water-damaged indoor carpeting be removed. You do not need to know all of the answers in how to get the school building to be healthier, but if you have specific ideas in mind, be sure to share them.

Know the Costs

With tight school budgets that seem to shrink every year, your local school or school district might immediately assume that any request for making a school healthier is going to involve great expense. Assure the school that this is not always the case and that, in fact, improvements can often be free or low-cost. Allowing teachers to open their windows to get fresh air inside the classroom is a completely free improvement to a school's indoor air quality. Caulking cracks in the school's foundation to prevent rodents from entering is a cheaper alternative to pesticides and pest-control services. Switching to greener cleaners might cost the same as harsh toxic brands, or it might cost less and end up saving the school money in the long run.

When suggesting alternatives, it is always helpful to find schools that have had the same problems and treated them effectively. An Internet search will allow you to find news reports and articles on specific schools and school systems across the country and the healthy changes that they have implemented. If financial facts and figures are included, especially if the healthy change is a no-cost or cost-saving alternative, use that information to encourage administration that healthy environmental changes are well within the budget and might actually help the school to save money.

Outfit Your Child

Until positive changes are made within the school, you might need to supply your child with healthy alternatives. Whether you do it on your own or join forces with other parents in the classroom or school, supplying your child with items to use at school is the only way that you know for sure what your child is exposed to throughout the day. Decide what the hazard is and how you can come up with a healthy solution, if possible. For example, if questionable water quality is an issue, give your child bottles of water or other healthy drinks to consume during school. If harsh chemical cleaners are leading to poor indoor air quality, ask the teacher if you can supply green cleaners to be used in the classroom instead. Ask if you can donate several hardy plants to each classroom that your child spends time in to naturally filter the indoor air and remove pollutants.

You might believe that you should not have to pay for any health improvements at the school, but unfortunately, that might have to be the case, especially with schools facing budget cutbacks every year. Talk with your child's teachers and ask if there are any changes that are not being made because of lack of money. If you or a group of parents can purchase a new air filter, cleaning products, water filters, etc., the investment in your child's health will be well worth it.

CHECKLIST FOR A HEALTHY SCHOOL

❑ Realize that there can be little regulation regarding the health of a school building. Once you know that there might not be many standards in place regarding mold exposure, indoor air quality, and use of pesticides, you might be more encouraged to start looking into the health of your child's specific school.

❏ Partner with fellow parents and teachers to make positive changes. The more people who are concerned about children's health, the more likely there will be a positive change.

❏ Use extensive online resources to reach out to your child's school. You don't need to research everything on your own. Many nonprofit organizations will happily supply the information to help you fight for health at school.

❏ If necessary, supply your child with healthier products. Sometimes it might be necessary to give your child supplies from home that you feel are healthier than what the school will supply.

APPENDIX A

Further Reading

Books

Hunter, Linda Mason, and Mikki Halpin. *Green Clean: The Environmentally Sound Guide to Cleaning Your Home.* (New York, NY: DK Melcher Media, 2005).

Lansky, Vicki. *Baking Soda: Over 500 Fabulous, Fun, and Frugal Uses You've Probably Never Thought Of.* (Deephaven, MN: Book Peddlers, 2003).

Lansky, Vicki. *Vinegar: Over 400 Various, Versatile, and Very Good Uses You've Probably Never Thought Of.* (Deephaven, MN: Book Peddlers, 2003).

Lifton, Bernice. *Bug Busters: Poison-Free Pest Controls for Your House & Garden.* (Garden City Park, NY: Square One Publishers, 2005).

Lutz, Kim, and Megan Hart. *The Everything Organic Cooking for Baby and Toddler Book: 300 Naturally Delicious Recipes to Get Your Child Off to a Healthy Start.* (Avon, MA: Adams Media, 2008).

Malkan, Stacy. *Not Just a Pretty Face: The Ugly Side of the Beauty Industry.* (Gabriola Island, BC, Canada: New Society Publishers, 2007).

O'Connor, Siobhan, and Alexandra Spunt. *No More Dirty Looks: The Truth about Your Beauty Products—and the Ultimate Guide to Safe and Clean Cosmetics.* (Cambridge, MA: Da Capo Lifelong Books, 2010).

Pitcairn, Richard. *Dr. Pitcairn's New Complete Guide to Natural Health for Dogs and Cats.* (Emmaus, PA: Rodale Books, 2005).

Schapiro, Mark. *Exposed: The Toxic Chemistry of Everyday Products and What's at Stake for American Power.* (White River Junction, VT: Chelsea Green Publishing, 2009).

Smith, Rick, and Bruce Lourie. *Slow Death by Rubber Duck.* (Berkeley, CA: Counterpoint, 2010).

Taggart, Jennifer. *Smart Mama's Green Guide: Simple Steps to Reduce Your Child's Toxic Chemical Exposure.* (Boston, MA: Center Street, 2009).

Tukey, Paul. *The Organic Lawn Care Manual: A Natural, Low-Maintenance System for a Beautiful, Safe Lawn.* (North Adams, MA: Storey Publishing, 2007).

Winter, Ruth. *A Consumer's Dictionary of Cosmetic Ingredients.* (New York, NY: Three Rivers Press, 2009).

Wolverton, B. C. *How to Grow Fresh Air: 50 House Plants That Purify Your Home or Office.* (New York, NY: Penguin, 1997).

Websites

Beauty Is Wellness
Information and product reviews on natural and chemical-free beauty products.
www.beautyiswellness.com

The Campaign for Safe Cosmetics
A coalition of organizations and companies that work to reform the cosmetic industry and encourage the elimination of dangerous chemicals from personal care products.
www.safecosmetics.org

Care2

A wealth of advice on how to live a healthier, greener lifestyle and support socially responsible causes. *www.care2.com*

Get Green Be Well

Covers all aspects of living a greener life to live a healthier life, including travel, product reviews, gardening, beauty, and home. *www.getgreenbewell.com*

The Smart Mama

Founded by a mother and environmental lawyer, this site gives the gritty details of product testing and chemical exposures in everyday products and calls out companies for bogus marketing claims. *www.thesmartmama.com*

Phone Applications

Dirty Dozen

Lists the produce items with the highest and least amount of pesticides to help you choose when to pay more for organics. *www.ewg.org/foodnews/guide*

EWG Sunscreen Buyer's Guide

Offers analysis on the safety of more than 1,700 sunscreen products. *www.ewg.org/iPhone_App_For_Sunscreens*

GoodGuide mobile

Search more than 120,000 entries to find safe, healthy, and sustainable products while you shop. *www.goodguide.com/about/mobile*

Healthy Child Healthy World Pocket Guides

A collection of mini-guides on how to live a healthier life, including green cleaning, avoiding chemicals in personal care products, safer plastics, and healthy baby products. *http://healthychild.org/live-healthy/pocket_guides*

Label Lookup

Do not be confused by label claims anymore. Look up a marketing claim with this app and find out exactly what it means. *http://itunes.apple.com/us/app/label-lookup/ id340129104?mt=8*

Lady Bird Johnson Wildflower Center

A database of native plants and wildflowers for your landscaping projects. *www.wildflower.org/mobile*

Organizations That Support a Healthy Home

American Lung Association
1301 Pennsylvania Ave. NW, Suite 800
Washington, DC 20004
1-800-548-8252
www.lungusa.org

The American Lung Association fights to save lives by preventing lung diseases and educating the public on lung health hazards, including environmental health concerns and poor indoor air quality.

Beyond Pesticides
701 E St. SE, Suite 200
Washington, DC 20003
(202) 543-5450
www.beyondpesticides.org

Beyond Pesticides' goal is to create a world without the harmful use of toxic pesticides. The nonprofit organization offers a wealth of information on all forms of pesticides, including lawn and garden, as well as antibacterials, organic foods, genetic engineering, and healthy schools and hospitals.

Environmental Working Group
1436 U St. NW, Suite 100
Washington, DC 20009
(202) 667-6982
www.ewg.org

A nonprofit organization that strives to protect public health and the environment by launching investigations into the health and safety of consumer products, as well as lobbying politicians and industry for policy changes. EWG is well known for their annual Dirty Dozen list, an updated list that comes out each year highlighting the produce crops of the previous year that had the highest and lowest amounts of pesticides.

Healthy Building Network
2001 S. Street NW, Suite 570
Washington, DC 20009
(877) 974-2767
www.healthybuilding.net

The Healthy Building Network focuses on promoting building materials that have the best environmental, health, and social justice impacts.

Healthy Child Healthy World
12300 Wilshire Blvd., Suite 320
Los Angeles, CA 90025
(310) 820-2030
www.healthychild.org

A nonprofit whose mission is to empower parents to protect their children from harmful chemicals. Healthy Child Healthy World offers online tutorials, healthy home party kits, apps, and mini-guides that frame the complex challenges of creating a chemical-free environment for children into easily understood terms and solutions.

Healthy Schools Network

110 Maryland Ave. NE, Suite 505
Washington, DC 20002
(202) 543-7555
www.healthyschools.org

A nonprofit organization that strives to change the policies of environmental health in schools and to create healthier environments for learning.

National Lead Information Center

422 South Clinton Ave.
Rochester, NY 14620
(800) 424-5323
www.epa.gov/lead/pubs/nlic.htm

With funding from the EPA and the Department of Housing and Urban Development, the National Lead Information Center provides the public with education materials and answers questions via phone, mail, e-mail, and fax.

Safe Lawns Foundation

9 Cole St.
Falmouth, ME 04105
(207) 252-0869
www.safelawns.org

A coalition of nonprofit organizations and businesses that work together to educate the public about environmentally responsible lawn care. More than twenty videos on the website demonstrate easy organic lawn techniques to reduce your chemical exposure.

U.S. Environmental Protection Agency

Ariel Rios Building, 1200 Pennsylvania Ave. NW
Washington, DC 20460
(202) 272-0167
www.epa.gov

Governmental agency empowered to protect human health and the environment. The EPA develops and enforces regulations of health and safety standards that affect all Americans, both at home and in work settings.

Index

We Have
EVERYTHING®
on Anything!

With more than 19 million copies sold, the Everything® series has become one of America's favorite resources for solving problems, learning new skills, and organizing lives. Our brand is not only recognizable—it's also welcomed.

The series is a hand-in-hand partner for people who are ready to tackle new subjects—like you!

For more information on the Everything® series, please visit *www.adamsmedia.com*

The Everything® list spans a wide range of subjects, with more than 500 titles covering 25 different categories:

Business	History	Reference
Careers	Home Improvement	Religion
Children's Storybooks	Everything Kids	Self-Help
Computers	Languages	Sports & Fitness
Cooking	Music	Travel
Crafts and Hobbies	New Age	Wedding
Education/Schools	Parenting	Writing
Games and Puzzles	Personal Finance	
Health	Pets	